HIV and Psychological Issues

Volume 3

HIV and Psychological Issues

Annual Special Issue

December, 2015

Chief Editor (IJIP)

Prof. Suresh M. Makvana, PhD

Guest Chief Editor (Special Issue)

Dr. Hitesh H. Patel, MBBS, DGO

Managing Editor

Ankit P. Patel, Clinical Psychology

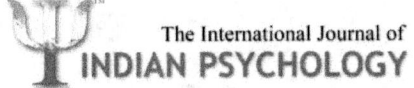

The International Journal of
INDIAN PSYCHOLOGY

HIV and Psychological Issues
By IJIP

-

ISBN-13: 978-1519557476
ISBN-10: 1519557477
Amazon Catalog: 5899960
Paperback
Price $ 10.70 USD (for World)
Edition: 2015

***

Exclusive Publisher and Distributor
Amazon, Inc
P.O. BOX 81226 Seattle,
WA 98108 USA
Contact: 206.266.4064
info@amazon.com
www.amazon.com
***
In Association with
The International Journal of Indian Psychology
88, Patel Street, Navamuvada,
Lunawada, Gujarat, India-389230
Contact: 76988 26988
journal@ijip.in
www.ijip.in

Edited in India
Printed in the USA

to,
HIV Patients…

Message from Editor in- Chief (IJIP)

We know that full name of AIDS is Acquired Immune Deficiency Syndrome. We also know that it happens due to HIV (Human Immunodeficiency Virus). Moreover, we also know that, HIV destroys resisting power of a person against disease, affecting Immune system of a person. Even knowing all these, AIDS is increasing day by day. What can be the reason of it? Perhaps its reason may be sexuality, because sexuality is a most weakness of a person. A person may be expert in any field, but when the point of sexuality comes, every person seems standing in the same line. Sex without any restriction attracts to every person, but due to this weakness, demon of AIDS is standing against our generation and we are helpless.

All the world celebrates 1st December as a "World AIDS Day." Glory of this day resides in, to aware of dangerous disease like AIDS and to prevent it. The International Journal of Indian Psychology has organized to bring out Annual Special Issue on HIV and psychological Issues giving its contribution in this benevolence work in which a try has been done to publish all research papers presented to them in free publishing policy.

We express here all the authors of these research papers who have submitted their articles/ papers to support this issue and we cannot forget who have supported us commercially. We recall here all indexing partners, universities and organization who are connected with us.

We hope that, this issue will play its role in relation with AIDS.

Dr. Suresh Makwana, PhD

Prof. Dept. of Psychology,

Sardar Patel University, Vallbh Vidyanagar

Message from Chief Editor (Special Issue)

AIDS is a mirror showing boundary, limitation or failure of medical science. From 1981 (in the United States) thousands of people have been victimized of this disease. According to a report of 2014, 1.2 million people had been died due to HIV and other 36.9 million people are living with HIV. Danger of HIV infection is Blood transfusion 90% , Childbirth (to child) 25%, Needle-sharing injection drug use 0.67%, Percutaneous needle stick 0.30%, Receptive anal intercourse 0.04–3.0%, Insertive anal intercourse 0.03%, Receptive penile-vaginal intercourse 0.05–0.30%, Insertive penile-vaginal intercourse 0.01–0.38%, Receptive oral intercourse 0–0.04% , Insertive oral intercourse 0–0.005%.

When HIV virus enters in the body of a person, his/her CD4+T lymphocyte becomes very less within 3 to 10 weeks (200 to 100 cell/mm^3), against it, HIV RNA increase very fast (10^6 to 10^7 per mL of plasma).

Many people know AIDS as a disease but it is not a disease, but it is a position (state or stage) of body. It is such a condition in which his/her resisting power decreases gradually and body of a person becomes colony for more than one disease ((Immune system defends the body, White blood cells (WBCs) are the most important part of this immune system, WBCs fight and destroy bacteria, fungi and viruses that enter the body). It includes from general disease like, fever, cold to dangerous diseases like T.B. (tuberculosis) and Brain Hemerage.

I welcome heartily to try done by IJIP under the world AIDS Day. IJIP has joined AIDS with Psychology and joined psychological factors in the direction of AIDS which is receptible and I have honor of becoming a part of it. I am thankful to team of IJIP who have considered me worthy for it. I am thankful to Prof. (Dr.) Suresh Makwana sir, Chief Editor and also Ankit Patel, Managing Editor of IJIP who have made done such good fortune to me. Many congratulations to authors of all research papers published in special issue. Really it was a happier experience for me to work with creative minds of psychology. I hope, such experience, would be got frequently by IJIP.

Dr. Hitesh Patel, M.B.B.S., D.G.O

Chief Surgeon, Vardan Hospital, Dist. Dahod

Index of Volume 3, HIV and Psychological Issues

Disclaimer

The International Journal of Indian Psychology (IJIP) provides platform for researchers to publish and discuss their original research and review work. IJIP cannot be held responsible for views, opinions and written statements of researchers published in the journal. IJIP strongly condemn and discourage practice of plagiarism.

HIV and Liver Diseases

Prof. Suresh Makvana[1], Ankit Patel[2]

Keywords: *HIV/AIDS, Liver Disease*

Coinfection with hepatitis B virus (HBV) and HIV is common, with 70-90% of HIV-infected individuals in the United States having evidence of past or active infection with HBV. Factors affecting the prevalence of chronic HBV include age at time of infection and mode of acquisition, which vary geographically. In the United States and Western Europe, HBV often is acquired in adolescence or adulthood via sexual contact or injection drug use. Although spontaneous clearance of HBV acquired in adulthood occurs in >90% of immunocompetent individuals, HIV-infected persons are half as likely as HIV-uninfected persons to spontaneously clear HBV. Therefore, chronic HBV infection occurs in 5-10% of HIV-infected individuals who are exposed to HBV, a rate 10 times higher than that for the general population. In the United States, HIV/HBV coinfection rates are highest among men who have sex with men (MSM) and injection drug users. In contrast, in Asia and sub-Saharan Africa, where vertical and early childhood exposure are the most common modes of transmission, respectively, and overall HBV prevalence is higher, the prevalence of HBV among HIV-infected individuals also is higher, at an estimated 20-30%.

HBV is a DNA virus that forms stable circular covalently closed (ccc) DNA that can persist in the liver indefinitely. Individuals with evidence of past infection (core antibody positivity) are at risk of HBV reactivation, particularly in the setting of severe immunocompromise, prolonged steroid use, or chemotherapy. There

[1](PhD) Professor, Dept. of Psychology, Sardar Patel University, Vallbh Vidyanagar
[2] Clinical Psychology, Sardar Patel University, Vallbh Vidyanagar

are 8 genotypes of HBV. Genotype G may be predictive of more severe fibrosis in HIV-coinfected patients, and genotypes C and D may be more responsive to interferon. However, in general, knowledge of the HBV genotype is not consistently associated with a response to nucleoside therapy and therefore is not particularly useful in clinical care of HIV/HBV coinfection, as nucleosides are the mainstays of HBV treatment.

ACUTE AND CHRONIC HEPATITIS B

When a person is first infected with the hepatitis B virus, this is called an acute infection. A person may not have any symptoms or s/he could become seriously ill. Most adults will recover and get rid of the virus without any problems. If the virus remains in the blood for more than six months, then a person is diagnosed as having a *chronic infection.*

Unfortunately, this is not true for infants and young children *90% of infants and up to 50% of young children infected with hepatitis B will not get rid of the virus and will develop a chronic infection.* A smaller number of infected adults (5-10%) will also become chronically infected with hepatitis B.

Epidemiology

The leading cause of chronic liver disease and is transmitted through sexual contact and IV drug use. HIV infection is associated with an inceased risk developing hepatitis B. Patients with chronic hepatitis B infection are at increased risk of hepatocelluar carcinoma.

Clinical features

Acute infection may present with fatigue, right upper quadrant abdominal pain, nausea, vomiting, fever, arthralgia and jaundice. The disease may remain asymptomatic until the onset of end-stage liver disease (ESLD) which is heralded by ascites, coagulopathy, palmar erythema, jaundice, hepatospenomegaly, variceal bleeding or encephalopathy. There may also be polyarteritis nodosa, glomerulonephritis and vasculitis.

Diagnosis

Test for hepatitis B surface antigen (HBsAg) antibody to hepatitis B core antigen (anti-HBc) and antibody to hepatitis B surface antigen (anti-HBs) will indentify the majority of patients. It will also determine which individuals require vaccination. A chronic stage is said to occur when HBsAg is present for more than six months. Once detected, the severity of the liver disease must be followed with assessment of alanine transaminase (ALT) serum albumin, prothrombin time, platelet count, and completed blood count and bilirubin levels. Patients should also be monitored every six months with alpha-fetoprotein levels and ultrasound of the liver, especially if they are older than 45 years, alcoholic, have cirrhosis or have a family history of chronic liver disease. Liver biopsy should be done to assess the grade and stage of liver disease. Transient elevation of enzymes can occur as a result of the hepatotoxicity of various drugs used in HAART. It may also occur as a result of concomitant infection with hepatitis A, hepatitis C or hepatitis delta virus.

Treatment

Patient should avoid alcohol. All their contacts-sexual, household and needle sharing need to be immunized. If the person also develops hepatitis A, it is likely to be fulminant and therefore active immunization with two doses of hepatitis A vaccine should be administered before the CD4 count falls to <200 cells/mm^3.

Antiviral treatment is advised if there is actively replicating virus in the blood, indicated by a positive hepatitis B core antigen (HBcAg) or HBV DNA levels>10^5 copies/ml and a raised ALT level that is twice the normal. Pegylated interferon (PEN IFN) alpha 2,5-10 MU can be given thrice a week subcutaneously (SC) for 16-24 weeks. If the patient is HAART-naïve, lamivudine is the preferred drug along with other ARV drugs. Adefovir dipivoxil 10 mg OD can be used in patients who do not require HAART. Tenofovir 300 mg OD can also be used. Emtricitabine 200 mg OD is also active against replication of the hepatitis B virus. If the patient is infected with HBV, HBC, and HIV-1, starting HAART should be the first priority. If HAART is not required then treatment for HBV should be considered first.

If ESLD develops I managed is the same way as in HIV negative individuals. IFN is contraindicated in ESLD. Liver transplantation can be done.

ACUTE AND CHRONIC HEPATITIS C

Epidemiology

Chronic Hepatitis C infection is caused by the single long-stranded RNA Hepatitis C virus. There are 6 genotypes and 50 subtypes. It is transmitted sexually, through infected blood products, needle-sharing and from mother to child. Cirrhosis sets in approximately 20 years after infection. The incidence of cirrhosis is higher in males, those>45 years and which concomitant alcoholism. Co-infection with HIV increases the rapidity of progression to ESLD.

Clinical Features

Patients may be asymptomatic or only mildly systemic so that acute infection is not recognized. There may be low-grade fever, fatigue, anorexia, right upper quadrant pain, nausea, vomiting, dark-coloured urine and frank jaundice. ALT and aspartate aminotransferase (AST) may be elevated. Serum cryoglobulins are present in 60% but may not cause symptoms. As liver disease progress, signs of portal hypertension may appear. There may be leukocytoclastic vasculitis and porphyria cutanea tarda. Fibrosing cholestatic Hepatitis might occur.

4

Diagnosis

Qualitative HCV RNA assay in the blood shows>50 copies/ml. A recombinant immunoblot assay (RIBA) can be performed if the HCV RNA is negative but the immunoassay for anti-HCV is positive. HCV viral load does not correlate with the degree of histological injury. Co-infected persons should be checked for other co-morbid liver conditions such as hepatocellular carcinoma by serum alfafetoprotein level and ultrasound examinations of the liver. ALT is the simplest and least expensive test to evaluate the activity of liver disease.

Treatment

All patients should be counseled to stop alcohol consumption. Fulminant hepatic failure occurs if there is co-infection with Hepatitis A. Hence, all patients should receive two doses of Hepatitis A vaccine before the CD4 count falls to <200 cell/mm^3. In addition, they should also receive Hepatitis B vaccine.

Treatment should be offered to patients as increased risk developing cirrhosis, patients with detectable plasma HCV RNA levels, and in those in whom liver biopsy shows inflammation, necrosis, portal or bridging fibrosis and elevated ALT levels. IFN alfa-2b 180 ᵘg weekly by subcutaneous injection plus ribavirin 600-1400 daily might eradicate HCV infection. Patients with unstable cardiopulmonary disease, anaemia unresponsive to erythropoietin or haemoglobinopathy can not be given ribavirin. The exact duration of treatment is not known but it is usually continued for 48 weeks. The critical CD4 level is 500 cells/mm^3 . Before it falls below this level, treatment for HCV should be started. If the CD4 count is already below this level, HAART should be started first. Liver transplantation is a primary treatment option.

Quantitative HCV RNA levels are the best estimate for treatment. A sustained virological response means an absence of detectable HCV

RNA (<50 IU/ml) after antiviral treatment for 2 weeks. Relapse is defined as the presence of detectable HCV RNA at the end of treatment.

HBV MEDICATIONS

Interferon

IFN is most effective for HBV treatment in patients with low levels of viremia and elevated transaminases, and it therefore may be less useful in patients with HIV/HBV coinfection than in those with HBV alone. In coinfected patients, IFN has been associated with lower rates of HBV treatment success and increased toxicity. It cannot be used for patients with decompensated cirrhosis and is not feasible as a long-term treatment, owing to adverse events and tolerability issues. There are no data for use of pegylated IFN in HIV/HBV coinfection.

Lamivudine and emtricitabine

These nucleoside analogues have similar activity against both HIV and HBV and they are commonly used components for HIV/HBV cotreatment. However, HIV-infected individuals should not receive 3TC or FTC monotherapy for HBV infection because resistance to those drugs develops in up to 90% of patients within 4 years of single-drug treatment. Resistance to 3TC and FTC is characterized by the development of mutations at HBV rtM204 (also known as YMDD mutations). Once 3TC resistance has developed, HBV medications such as telbivudine will no longer have activity against HBV, and agents such as entecavir may be less efficacious and more prone to development of HBV resistance. As with other agents that have activity against HIV, 3TC and FTC should be used only for patients on fully suppressive ART.

Entecavir

Entecavir is a guanosine analogue that appears to be more potent than either 3TC or adefovir. Entecavir resistance requires the development of several resistance mutations, including the rtM204 mutation that confers resistance to 3TC. In the presence of 3TC resistance, entecavir usually is active but may be more vulnerable to the development of further resistance (see above). Although entecavir initially was thought to have no anti-HIV activity, it has been demonstrated to select for the M184V mutation and should not be used in the absence of combination ART with full suppression of HIV viremia.

Telbivudine

Telbivudine is a thymidine analogue that also selects for the HBV rtM204 mutation, which leads to 3TC cross-resistance, and should not be used after 3TC or FTC failure. Telbivudine also may have anti-HIV activity and is not recommended for use without fully suppressive ART.

Adefovir

Adefovir initially was formulated as an anti-HIV agent but was not developed for that purpose, owing to an association with renal toxicity. At lower dosages, adefovir suppresses HBV replication but is less potent than telbivudine or tenofovir. Adefovir appears to be active against 3TC-resistant HBV. The use of adefovir largely has been supplanted in favor of treatment with tenofovir, a related but more potent agent and one that is active against HIV. At the dosage used to treat HBV, adefovir does not appear to be active against HIV and has not been associated convincingly with the development of HIV resistance mutations such as K65R. Adefovir is an option for HBV treatment in HIV-infected patients who decline or cannot take ART, but it should be used with caution.

Tenofovir

TDF is related to adefovir but it has more potent HBV activity and also can be used for HIV treatment. As with other agents that have activity against HIV, TDF should be used only for patients who are on fully suppressive ART. It usually is used in combination with 3TC or FTC as first-line therapy. HBV that is resistant to 3TC or adefovir can be treated effectively with TDF therapy.

REFERENCES

Akuta N, Kumada H. Influence of hepatitis B virus genotypes on the response to antiviral therapies. J Antimicrob Chemother. 2005 Feb;55(2):139-42.

Alter MJ. Epidemiology of viral hepatitis and HIV co-infection. J Hepatol. 2006;44(1 Suppl):S6-9.

Annie Luetkemeyer, (2010) Hepatitis B and HIV Coinfection, HIV InSite, October 2010

Benhamou Y, Bochet M, Thibault V, Calvez V, Fievet MH, Vig P, Gibbs CS, Brosgart C, Fry J, Namini H, Katlama C, Poynard T. Safety and efficacy of adefovir dipivoxil in patients co-infected with HIV-1 and lamivudine-resistant hepatitis B virus: an open-label pilot study. Lancet. 2001 Sep;358(9283):718-23

Benhamou Y, Bochet M, Thibault V, Di Martino V, Caumes E, Bricaire F, Opolon P, Katlama C, Poynard T.Long-term incidence of hepatitis B virus resistance to lamivudine in human immunodeficiency virus-infected patients. Hepatology. 1999 Nov;30(5):1302-6

Bodsworth N, Donovan B, Nightingale BN. The effect of concurrent human immunodeficiency virus infection on chronic hepatitis B: a study of 150 homosexual men. J Infect Dis. 1989 Oct;160(4):577-82

Di Martino V, Thevenot T, Colin JF, et al. Influence of HIV infection on the response to interferon therapy and the long-term outcome of chronic hepatitis B. Gastroenterology. 2002 Dec;123(6):1812-22.

Hepatitis B Foundation Cause for a cure, (2015), Acute vs. Chronic Hepatitis B, Reserved from http://www.hepb.org/patients/acute_vs_chronic.htm [12:33 Am, 8/11/2015]

Hoffmann CJ, Thio CL. Clinical implications of HIV and hepatitis B co-infection in Asia and Africa. Lancet Infect Dis. 2007 Jun;7(6):402-9.

Lacombe K, Massari V, Girard PM, et al. Major role of hepatitis B genotypes in liver fibrosis during coinfection with HIV. AIDS. 2006 Feb 14;20(3):419-27.

Low E, Cox A, Atkins M, et al. Telbivudine has activity against HIV. In: Program and abstracts of the 16th Conference on Retroviruses and Opportunistic Infections; February 8-11, 2009; Montreal. Abstract 813a.

McMahon MA, Jilek BL, Brennan TP, et al. The HBV drug entecavir--effects on HIV-1 replication and resistance. N Engl J Med. 2007 Jun 21;356(25):2614-21.

Naco (2007) Guidelines for Prevention and Management of Common Opportunistic Infection/Malignancies among HIV-Infected Adults and Adolescent; Ministry of Health and Family Welfare, Government of India, New Delhi

Núñez M, Pérez-Olmeda M, Díaz B, et al. Activity of tenofovir on hepatitis B virus replication in HIV-co-infected patients failing or partially responding to lamivudine. AIDS. 2002 Nov 22;16(17):2352-4.

Peters MG, Andersen J, Lynch P, et al; ACTG Protocol A5127 Team. Randomized controlled study of tenofovir and adefovir in chronic hepatitis B virus and HIV infection: ACTG A5127. Hepatology. 2006 Nov;44(5):1110-6.

Rodríguez-Méndez ML, González-Quintela A, Aguilera A, Barrio E. Prevalence, patterns, and course of past hepatitis B virus infection in intravenous drug users with HIV-1 infection. Am J Gastroenterol. 2000 May;95(5):1316-22

Scharschmidt BF, Held MJ, Hollander HH, Read AE, Lavine JE, Veereman G, McGuire RF, Thaler MM. Hepatitis B in patients with HIV infection: relationship to AIDS and patient survival. Ann Intern Med. 1992 Nov;117(10):837-8

Sheldon JA, Corral A, Rodés B, et al. Risk of selecting K65R in antiretroviral-naive HIV-infected individuals with chronic hepatitis B treated with adefovir. AIDS. 2005 Nov 18;19(17):2036-8.

Sherman M, Yurdaydin C, Sollano J, et al; AI463026 BEHoLD Study Group. Entecavir for treatment of lamivudine-refractory, HBeAg-positive chronic hepatitis B. Gastroenterology. 2006 Jun;130(7):2039-49.

Uneke CJ, Ogbu O, Inyama PU, et al. Prevalence of hepatitis-B surface antigen among blood donors and human immunodeficiency virus-infected patients in Jos, Nigeria. Mem Inst Oswaldo Cruz. 2005 Feb;100(1):13-6.

HIV and Neurological Diseases

Ankit Patel[3], Dr. Hitesh Patel[4]

Keywords: *HIV/AIDS, Neurological Disease*

Neurological manifestations are the initial symptoms of HIV infection in about 10 to 20% of patients. HIV enters the brain as early as two days after infection, and persists throughout the course of the disease. About 60% of those with advanced AIDS will have clinically evident Neurological dysfunction. Autopsy studies have demonstrated pathological abnormities of the nervous system in 75 to 90% of cases.

All levels of the nervous system may be involved and the degree of involvement is independent of the CD4 cell level, *follow to Tables*

Table 1, Neurological involvement in HIV infection

HIV related	OI related
• Acute aseptic meningitis • Chronic meningitis • HIV encephalopathy (AIDS dementia) • Vacuolar myelopathy • Peripheral neuropathy • Myopathy	• Cryptococcal meningitis • Cerebral toxoplasmosis • CMV retinitis and encephalitis • Progressive multifocal leukoencephalopathy (PML) • Primary CNS lymphoma • TB • Syphilis

[3] Clinical Psychology, Dept. of Psychology, Sardar Patel University, Vallbh Vidyanagar
[4] M.B.B.S., D.G.O, Chief Surgeon, Vardan Hospital, Dist. Dahod

Table 2, Neurological syndromes and opportunistic infection in AIDS (Aetiological Diagnoses)

Syndrome	Clinical features	Aetiology
Meningitis	Headache, fever, nausea, vomining, Altered consciousness	Cryptococcosis, syphilis, listeriosis, tuberculosis
Focal cerebral lesions	Headache, focal signs, convulsions	Toxoplasmosis, progressive multifocal leukoencephalopathy (PML), syphilis, cytomegalovirus
Encephalitis	Cognitive impairment, psychiatric, features, altered consciousness	Cytomegalovirus, herpes simplex, toxoplasmosis
Myelitis	Sensory disturbances, paraparesis, sphincter disturbance	Cytomegalovirus, herpes simplex, varicella zoster, syphilis, toxoplasmosis

Table 3, Conditions of the neurological system

Aetiology	Presenting signs and symptoms	Diagnostic (Laboratory, X-ray, etc)	Management and Treatment	Unique Features, Caveats
Toxoplasma gondii (toxoplasmosis)	*Clinical symptoms may evolve in less than 2 weeks* • Headache (Severe, Localized) • Fever • Confusion • Myalgia	Available at CT scan or MRI Toxoplasma IgG titre In a resource-constrained setting:	Treatment for acute phase >6 weeks Pyrimethamine 100-200 mg loading dose, than 50-100	Usually occurs when CD4 count <100 cells/mm^3 Clinical response in 1 week and MRI

	• Arthralgia • Focal neurogical defects such as seizures • Hemiparesis • Hemiplegia, • Crebellar, • Tremor, • Cranial nerve • Palsies, • Hemisensory loss, • Visual problems or blindness, • Personality changes and cognitive disorders	diagnosis based on clinical symptoms CT scan or MRI findings: multiple ring lesions in the cerebral hemispheres An HIV infected individual presenting with typical symptoms and normal cerebrospinal fluid (CSF) findings should be given treatment for toxoplasmosis. CSF values Protein: 10-150/ml WBC: 0-40 (monocytes) Blood: full blood count (FBC)	mg/day PO + folinic (or folic) acid 10 mg/day Po + sulfadiazine 1-2 g qid (Dexamethasone 4 mg PO or IV q 6 h for mass effect) OR TMP/SMX 5/25 mg/kg daily OR Clindamycin (600 mg tid) + Pyrimethamine 100 mg daily loading does Followed by 50 mg daily + folinic acid 10 mg daily *Maintenance* Preferred regimen: Suppressive therapy required after a patient has had toxoplasmos	response expected in 2 weeks Check blood picture regularly as the relatively high doses of drugs can lead to toxicities. Leucopenia, ombocytopenia and rash are common. Folinic acid reduces the risk of yelosuppresion During treatment, advise patients to maintain a high fluid intake and urine output. Secondary prophylaxia may be discontinued if free of toxoplasma encephalitis; and sustained CD4 + T

			is Pyrimetham ine 25-75 mg PO qid + folinic acid 10 mg qid + sulfadiazine 0.501.0 g PO qid (50% of acute dose) Give dapsone PO 100 mg once daily or clindamycin IV (or oral) 600 mg qid pr atovaquine 750 mg PO qid Eptoin 50-100 mg bid or tid or tegretol 100-200 mg bid or tid (to be started only if the patient has convulsions)	lymphocyte count of $>$ 200 cells/mm^3 for >6 months of ART
Mycobacter ial infection –M Tuberculosi s (TB meningitis)	• Gradual onset of headache and consciousness • Low-grade evening fever Night sweats • Weight loss • Neck stiffness	Lumbar puncture CSF microspcopy CSF may be cloudy		CD4<350 cells/mm^3 Up to 10% of AIDS patient who present with TB show involvemen

	and positive Kernig sigh • Cranial nerve palsies from exudate around base of the brain			t of the meninges. This results from rupture of a cerebral tuberculoma or is blood-borne. Always exclude cryptococcal meningitis by CFS microscopy (India ink stain)
Strept Pheumoniae, Neisseria, meningitides (meningitis)	• Fever • Headache • Stiff neck • Photophobia • Vomiting • Malaise • Irritability • Drowsiness • Coma • Symptoms tend to present within 1 week of infection. • May be preceded by a prodromal respiratory illness or score throat	CFS examination Full blood count Common finding; CFS shows increased pressure, cell count 100-10000/mm3 and decreased glucose <40 mg/dl or <50% of the simultaneous glucose blood level Gram stained smear of a spun sediment of CSF can reveal the	Penicillin (24 million units daily in divided doses every 2 to 3 hours) OR ampicillin (12 g daily in divided doses every 2-3 hours) OR chloramphenicol (4-6 g IV/day) Treatment should be continued for 10-14 days. Crystalline penicillin 2-3 mega units and chloramphe	Often encountered during late stages of HIV disease. Prompt diagnosis and aggressive management and treatment ensure a quick recovery.

			aetiological agent	nicol 500-700/750 mg 6 hourly for 10-14 days	
Cryptococc us neoformans (**cryptococc al meningitis**)	• Presentation usually nonspecific at onset, which may be true for > 1 month • Protracted headache and fever may be the only signs • Nausea, vomiting and stiff neck may be absent and focal neurological signs uncommon. • Extraneural symptoms include skin lesions, pneumonitis, pleural effusion and retinitis • Fever, malaise and nuchal pain signify a worse prognosis, and nausea, vomiting and altered mental status occur in the terminal stages		CSF values: Protein 30-150 mg/dl WBC: 0-100 (monocytes) Glucose decreased: 50-70 mg/dl Culture positive: 95-100% India ink positive: 60-80% Crypt Ag nearly 100% sensitive and specific India ink staining of spinal fluid Test spinal fluid and/or serum for cryptococcal antigen	Preferred regimen: Amphoterici n B 0.7 mg/kg/day IV + flucy-tosine 100 mg/kg/day POx 14 days, followed by fluconazole 400 mg/day x 8-10 weeks Finally, maintenance therapy with fluconazole 200 mg/day for life Alternate regimen: Amphoterici n B 0.7 mg/ kg/day IV + flucytosine 100 mg/kg/day POx 14 days followed by itraconazole 200 mg bid for 8 weeks Fluconazole 400 mg/day PO x 8 weeks,follo wed by 200 mg once	If untreated, it is slowly progressive and ultimately fatal. It occurs most often in patients with a CD4 count <100 cells/mm^3 Headache is secondary to fungal accumulati on, so the headache increases gradually overtime, goes away and then comes back and is harder to get rid of. Then it becomes continuous, and this is what the patient reports Repeated LP might be indicated as

				daily Itraconazole 200 mg PO tid x 3 days, then 200 mg PO bid x 8 weeks after initial treatment with amphotericin Fluconazole 400 mg/day PO + flucytosine 100 mg/kg/day PO	adjunctive therapy among patients with increased intracranial pressure Discontinuation of antifungal therapy can be considered among patients who remain asymptomatic, with CD4+T-lymphocyte count>100-200 cells/mm3 for >6 months
Cytomegalovirus (CMV)		• Fever ± delirium, lethargy, disorientation, malaise. Headache most common • Stiff neck, photophobia, cranial nerve deficits less common • No focal • Neurological deficits • Gastrointestinal symptoms: diarrhoea, colitis,	Retinal exam to check for changes Consult an ophthalmologist. CMV retinitis, characterized by creamy yellow white, haemorrhagic, full-thickness retinal opacification, which can	Foscarnet 60 mg/kg IV q8h or 90 mg/kg IV q12h x 14-21 days; ganciclovir 5 mg/kg IV bid x 14-21 days, then valganciclovir 900 mg PO qid Patients without immune recovery will need to be on	Evolution <2 weeks CD4 count <100 cells/mm^3 Although any part of the retina may be involved, there is a predilection for the posterior pole; involvement of the optic nerve

	oesophageal ulceration appear in 12-15% of patients • Respiratory symptoms, i.e. pneumonitis, present in - 1%	cause visual loss and lead to blindness if untreated; patient may be asymptomatic or complain of floaters, diminished acuity or visual field defects. Retinal detachment if disease is extensive UGI endoscopy when indicated	maintenance therapy lifelong for retinitis Extraocular: ganciclovir and/or foscarnet	head and macular region is common Treatment is very expensive and usually not available. CMV management needs special care. Therefore, early referral is essential
Progressive multifocal leukoencephalopathy (PML)	• Afebrile, alert, no headache • Progressively impaired speech, vision, motor function • Cranial nerve deficits and cortical blindness • Cognition affected relatively late	CT brain scan may be normal or remarkable for areas of diminished density or demyelination (deterioration of the covering of the nerve) PCR of CSF for detection of the James Canyon (JC) virus JC virus PCR positive in about 60% of cases Differential diagnosis:	There is no treatment for this illness ART can improve symptoms and prolong life	An end-stage complication of HIV, caused by the JC virus PML is rare in the general community, but relatively common in HIV infection (affecting 4% of all AIDS patients). Routine testing for HIV should be

		Toxoplasmosis, primary CNS lymphoma Definitive diagnosis is by brain biopsy (if available)		considered for any patient with PML. Evolution: weeks to months Usually occurs when CD4 count <100 cells/ mm^3
Primary CNS lymphoma	• Disease • progresses slowly over a few weeks • Afebrile; headache • Focal and multifocal neurological deficits (confusion, hemiplegia, seizures) • Mental status change (60%, personality or behavioural • Seizures (15%)	CT scan/MRI Location: preventricular in one or more sites Prominent oedema, irregular and solid on enhancement CSF: Normal—30-50% Protein—10-150/ml WBC—0-100 (monocytes) Cytology positive in <5% Suspect when toxoplasma IgG is negative or there is failure to respond to empirical treatment for toxoplasmosis	There is no cytotoxic chemotherapy for this disease. Irradiation can help some patients, but is considered palliative Corticosteroids can also help some patients	Primary CNS lymphoma is rare in the general community, but affects about 2% of AIDS patients Survival after diagnosis is usually limited (a few months only). Typical end-stage complication of HIV disease Evolution: 2-8 weeks Usually occurs when CD4 count <100 cells/ mm^3

| AIDS dementia complex (ADC) HIV-associated dementia [HAD] | • In up to 10% of patients, it is the first manifestation of HIV disease.
• Afebrile; general lethargy
• Triad of cognitive, motor and behavioural dysfunction
• Early:
• concentration and memory deficits,
• inattention, motor incoordination, ataxia, depression, emotional lability
• Late: global dementia, paraplegia, mutism
The frequency in all patients is 10-15% | Neuropsychological tests show subcortical dementia Mini-mental examinations not very sensitive | Possible benefit from antiretroviral regimens with agents that penetrate the

CNS (AZT, d4T, ABC, nevirapine)

Benefit of AZT at higher dose for mild or moderately severe cases is established; monitor therapy with neurocognitive tests

Anecdotal experience indicates response to ART, if started early Sedation for those who are agitated and aggressive —use smaller doses initially to avoid oversedation Close | Prevalence increases with improvement in general management of various OIs because patients live long enough to develop severe immune suppression. Patients present with a demeanour similar to Parkinson disease and may even be misdiagnosed as such |

			monitoring: to prevent self-harm to ensure adequate nutrition to diagnose and treat Ols early	

Aseptic meningitis

It may occur as one of the manifestations of acute HIV syndrome. The onset may be several weeks after the other manifestations of the acute HIV syndrome. There may be retro-orbital pain, confusion, irritability, polyneuropathy, polyradiculopathy, facial palsy and weakness. Seizures and Guillain-Barre syndrome may occur. HIV can be demonstrated and cultured in the CSF but not in the blood. Treatment is supportive.

Acute bacterial meningitis

Acute bacterial meningitis occurs with equal frequency in HIV-infected and -uninfected persons. Common organisms include S. pneumoniae, H. influenzae and N. meningitides. Jhe symptoms and signs include fever, headache, stiff neck, photophobia, vomiting, malaise, irritability, drowsiness and coma. Symptoms tend to present within one week of infection, and may be preceded by a prodromal respiratory illness or sore throat. On examination, the CSF shows increased pressure, a high cell count (100-10 000/mm^3), increased protein (>100 mg/dl) and decreased glucose (<40 mg/dl or <50% of the simultaneous glucose blood level). A Gram- stained smear of spun sediment of the CSF may reveal the aetiological agent. A full blood count should also be done. Where available, CT scan or MRI may be performed to evaluate focal neurological deficits. Specific treatment depends on the aetiological agent.

CRYPTOCOCCAL MENINGITIS

It is caused by *Cryptococcus neoformans* var *neoformans*. It is the most common fungal meningitis in AIDS and affects about 10%.The majority of cases are seen when the CD4+ counts are <50 cells/mm^3. It commonly presents as a subacute meningitis or meningoencephalitis with fever, malaise and headache. Classical symptoms and signs such as neck stiffness or photophobia occurs only in one-fourth to one-third of AIDS patients. Some patients may present with encephalopathic symptoms such as lethargy, altered mentation, personality changes and memory loss. Some patients have disseminated disease without concurrent meningitis. Approximately half of them have pulmonary involvement. Skin lesions may be seen.

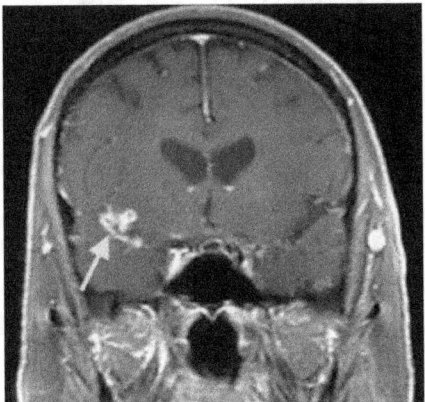

Figure 1; MR angiography of large vessel stenosis after cryptococcal meningitis

DIAGNOSIS

Analysis of the CSF usually shows mildly raised protein, normal or slightly low glucose, with an increased white cell count (5-100 cells: predominantly mononuclear lymphocytes).The opening pressure of the CSF is elevated. India ink staining demonstrates the organism. Culture of the CSF grows *Cryptococcus*. Up to 75% of those with HIV-associated cryptococcal meningitis have positive fungal blood cultures. Serum cryptococcal antigen might be useful in making an initial diagnosis.

Diagnosis is said to be *confirmed when Cryptococcus* is identified in the CSF or CNS tissue by positive culture or histopathology.

Diagnosis is said to be proboble in the presence of:
- Compatible clinical syndrome that includes fever and one or more of the following signs or symptoms of meningitis: headache, altered mental status, stiff neck and/or photophobia, seizures and/or focal deficits.
- Positive serum cryptococcal antigen
- Specific antifungal therapy initiated or recommended.
- Diagnosis is considered *possible* when:
    - There is a compatible clinical syndrome that includes fever and one or more of the following signs or symptoms of meningitis: headache, altered mental status, stiff neck and/or photophobia, seizures and/ or focal deficits, and
    - Specific antifungal therapy initiated or recommended.

TREATMENT
Untreated, cryptococcal meningitis is fatal. The recommended initial treatment for acute disease is amphotericin B for 2 weeks, followed by fluconazole alone for an additional 8 weeks. This approach has a mortality of <10% and a mycological response of 70%. If new symptoms or clinical findings occur after 2 weeks of treatment, a repeat LP should be performed. Serial measurement of CSF cryptococcal antigen might be useful but require repeated LPs and is not routinely recommended. Patients treated with amphotericin B should be monitored for dose-dependent nephrotoxicity and electrolyte disturbances.

Lipid formulations of amphotericin B are fairly effective in doses of 4 mg/kg daily. However, under the national programme, non-lipid formulations of amphotericin B are provided. Combination therapy with fluconazole (400-800 mg/daily) and flucytosine is also effective for treating AIDS-associated cryptococcal meningitis but the latter is not available in India.

Primary therapy

Acute - Induction: Amphotericin B (0.7 mg/kg/d) ± 5- flucytosine 25 mg/kg qid x 14 days Consolidation: Fluconazole 400 mg/day for 8-10 weeks or until the CSF is sterile.

Maintenance: Fluconazole 200 mg/day lifelong (stop when the CD4+ count is >200 cells/mm^3 for 3 months)

Lumbar puncture: Repeated LPs are needed if the CSF opening pressure is >250 mmH$_2$O.The initial LP should reduce the opening pressure by 50%. Daily LPs are needed to maintain the opening pressure at <200 mm CSF. LP may be stopped once the opening pressure has been normal for several consecutive days. CSF shunting should be considered when daily LPs are no longer tolerated or when the signs and symptoms of cerebral oedema are not relieved. Acetazolamide has no role in reducing the intracranial pressure.

Maintenance therapy

Without maintenance therapy, relapse occurs in 50-60% of patients within 6 months. Maintenance therapy is given with fluconazole at a dose of 200 mg daily lifelong or until the CD4+ count remains above 200 cells/ mm^3 for 3-6 months in a patient on HAART. Alternative therapy is possible with amphotericin B, voriconazole, and high-dose fluconazole + terbinafin.

Fluconazole has drug interactions with nevirapine used in HAART and leads to hepatotoxicity in 25% of patients receiving both drugs.

This combination has to be used with caution and with regular monitoring of liver function tests.

Failure of therapy

With maintenance therapy, relapses are uncommon and usually related to noncompliance. Rarely, drug resistance and drug interactions which lower fluconazole levels may be responsible. Monitoring serum cryptococcal antigen titres is not useful in predicting relapse.

CEREBRAL TOXOPLASMOSIS

It is caused by the protozoon *Toxoplasma gondii*. Although *T. gondii* usually causes encephalitis, it also causes disease in various organs including the eyes and lungs. Infection is acquired by contact with cats or birds, and eating undercooked meat, especially pork, lamb or venison. Encephalitis occurs from reactivation of latent cysts, and is most common among HIV-positive people with CD4 counts <50 cells/mm^3. Anti-*Toxoplasma* antibodies are not protective and only indicate prior infection.

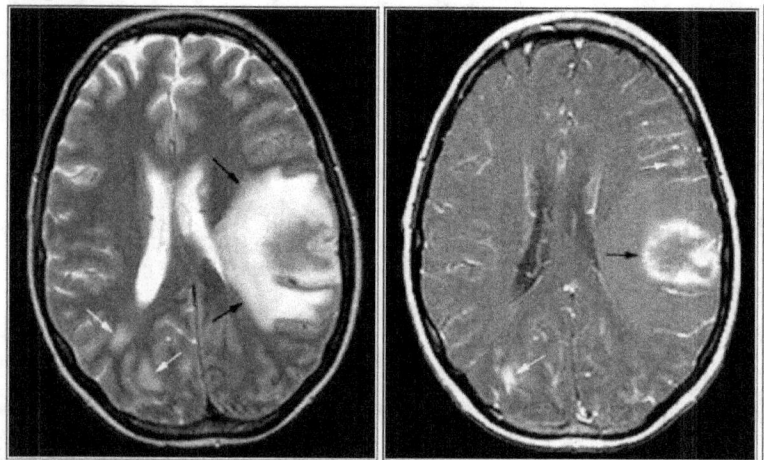

Figure 2, (Left) Axial T2-Weighted image shows a left temporal lobe mass with surrounding edema (black arrows) other small lesions are seen in right parietal lobe (white arrows)
Figure 3, (Right) Axial contrast T1-weighted image shows nodular and irregular ring enhancement (black arrows), small enhancing lesions are seen in bilateral cerebral hemispheres (white arrows)

CLINICAL FEATURES

Symptoms include headache, fever, confusion, progressive focal neurological deficits, seizures, abnormal behaviour, motor weakness and coma.

DIAGNOSIS

Serum IgG and IgM *anti-Toxoplasma* antibodies can be estimated, but do not indicate active disease. Polymerase chain reaction (PCR) tests have high specificity but low sensitivity. CT or MRI scans showing focal lesions may be helpful in making a diagnosis, although differentiation from other CNS diseases such as lymphoma may be difficult. Newer imaging devices such as positron emission tomography (PET) or single photon emission computed tomography (SPECT) scans may be more helpful, although more expensive. Stereotactic CT-guided brain biopsy is reserved for patients who fail to respond to therapy.

TREATMENT

If CNS toxoplasmosis is suspected, treatment should precede confirmation of diagnosis. Brain biopsy is required only if the patient does not respond to treatment. Biopsy may be required to diagnose toxoplasmosis of other tissues such as the lungs.

A combination of pyrimethamine, sulfadiazine and leucovorin is the recommended initial regimen. Pyrimethamine is started orally at a dose of 100-200 mg daily, followed by a lower dose. It penetrates the brain parenchyma even if there is no inflammation. Leucovorin contains folate, and decreases the haematological side-effects of pyrimethamine. Sulfadiazine is given orally four times a day at a dose of 4-8 g/day. Clindamycin or TMP-SMX can be used in case sulfadiazine is not available.

Other combnations used include: atovaquone + sulfadiazine; atovaquone + pyrimethamine + leucovorin; azithromycin +

pyrimethamine + leucovorin. Dapsone, 5-fluorouracil, clarithromycin, and minocycline have all been used with in various permutations and combinations.

Initially, high doses of these medications are given for 4-6 weeks followed by lower doses as maintenance therapy to prevent recurrence. Maintenance therapy can be discontinued in an asymptomatic patient on HAART with a CD4 count >200 cells/mm^3 for at least 6 months. It has to be restarted if the CD4 count falls or the MRI/CT shows persistent cerebral mass lesions.

Corticosteroids such as dexamethasone may help control inflammation of the brain in patients with focal neurological symptoms. However, they need to be used carefully, given that corticosteroids may precipitate other OIs. Anticonvulsants should be administered only if there is a history of seizures and should not be used prophylactically.

ADVERSE EVENTS
Pyrimethamine can cause rash, nausea and bone marrow suppression. Sulfadiazine and TMP-SMX can cause rash, fever, leucopenia, hepatitis, nausea, vomiting, diarrhoea, crystalluria, hepatotoxicity and *Clostridium difficile* colitis. Drug interactions between anticonvulsants and ART may necessitate adjustment of dosages.

PREVENTION
The best way to prevent toxoplasmosis is to avoid contact with *T. gondii*. Meats such as pork, lamb or venison should be well cooked. Precautions should be followed while handling cats and birds.

Daily TMP-SMX is the most effective regimen to prevent toxoplasmosis. For patients who are allergic, dapsone + pyrimethamine + folic acid once a week is a good alternative.

AIDS DEMENTIA COMPLEX (ADC)

ADC or HIV-associated dementia (HAD) is different from other OIs in that the disease is caused by the HIV itself, which enters the brain as early as two days after infection. HIV can then damage the nerve cells in the brain. ADC is more likely with CD4 counts <200 cells/mm^3. Between 20% and 35% of all HIV-positive people eventually develop ADC at CD4 counts of 100-200 cells/mm^3.

There is acquired and slowly progressive cognitive decline, motor and behavioural changes, and non-focal or diffuse CNS signs. Signs of early dementia include: trouble learning new things, difficulty remembering things that happened in the past, changes in behaviour, confusion and depression. Advanced dementia produces abnormalities of speech, balance, vision, gait, and loss of bladder control. It can also lead to mania (exaggerated feeling of well-being) or psychosis (loss of contact with reality).

DIAGNOSIS

ADC is a *diagnosis of exclusion*. The CSF findings are non-specific and CT/MRI shows only cerebral atrophy and ventricular dilatation. Several AIDS-related diseases such as toxoplasmosis, lymphoma and PML can cause symptoms similar to those of ADC.

TREATMENT

HAART is the most effective treatment and ARV regimens should include agents that penetrate the CNS (AZT, d4T, ABC, nevirapine). Even though HAART can treat the underlying cause, it may not effectively treat the symptoms, and may actually worsen them in some cases. Additional supportive treatment strategies may be needed in some cases. Sedation is required for those who are agitated and aggressive, with smaller initial doses to avoid over sedation. Close monitoring to prevent self-harm, adequate nutrition, early diagnosis and treatment of other OIs, and psychological support for caregivers are important accessories to therapy.

PRIMARY CNS LYMPHOMA

Primary CNS lymphoma is rare in the general community, but affects about 2% of HIV/AIDS patients. Survival after diagnosis is usually limited to a few months only. It is a typical end-stage complication of HIV disease. The disease evolves over 2-8 weeks. It usually occurs when the CD4 count is <100 cells/mm^3.

Disease progression occurs over a few weeks. Patients are afebrile, with headache and focal neurological deficits (confusion, hemiplegia, seizures). They may present with mental status changes (60%), and personality or behavioural changes. Seizures occur in 15%.

DIAGNOSIS

CT scan/MRI shows periventricular irregular lesions which appear solid on enhancement in one or more sites. There is prominent oedema. Lymphoma is suspected when the *Toxoplasma* IgG is negative or there is failure to respond to empirical treatment for toxoplasmosis. Neuropsychological tests show subcortical dementia. Mini-mental status examinations are not very sensitive. CSF analysis is normal in 30-50% of patients. The CSF cytology is positive for malignant cells in <5% of patients.

TREATMENT

There is no cytotoxic chemotherapy for this disease. Irradiation can help some patients, but is considered palliative. Corticosteroids can also help some patients.

PROGRESSIVE MULTIFOCAL LEUKOENCEPHALOPATHY (PML)

PML results from multifocal demyelination caused by the James Canyon (JC) virus. It is a neurological condition that progresses relatively rapidly over weeks to months with cognitive dysfunction, ataxia, aphasia, cranial nerve deficits, hemiparesis or quadriparesis, and eventually coma.

DIAGNOSIS

Typical CTscan findings include single or multiple hypodense, non-enhancing cerebral white matter lesions. Diagnosis is *confirmed* if histopathology or in situ hybridization from a brain biopsy or CSF PCR shows the JC virus.

Diagnosis is considered *probable* if the clinical presentation (subacute progressive focal neurological deficits including hemiparesis, field deficits, ataxia, or other abnormality referable to dysfunction of a specific brain region, and does not include cognitive impairment alone) and MRI findings are compatible with PML

Diagnosis is considered *possible* if the clinical presentation is consistent with PML, and focal lesions without mass effect or enhancement are seen on CT or MRI of brain.

TREATMENT

HAART is the only effective treatment and many studies have used even more than three drugs in HAART (mega HAART) but the current recommendation is triple-drug ART only.

CYTOMEGALOVIRUS INFECTION

Cytomegalovirus (CMV) or herpes virus type 4 is a double-stranded DNA virus. Infection is common, and latency follows infection. Almost all homosexual or bisexual men and more than 75% of all HIV-infected people carry the virus. A small percentage with severely compromised immune systems actually develops CMV disease when immunosuppressant reactivates inherent CMV to cause disseminated or localized end- organ disease. Around 30% of patients with AIDS develop CMV retinitis sometime between the diagnosis of AIDS and death.

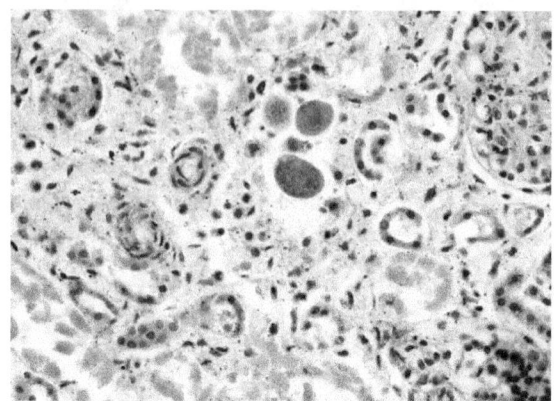

Figure 4, Cytomegalovirus Infection

CLINICAL MANIFESTATIONS

Retinitis is the most common manifestation. CMV retinitis usually occurs unilaterally, but may be bilateral. Peripheral retinitis might be asymptomatic, or may present with floaters, scotomata or peripheral visual field defects. Central retinal lesions or lesions impinging on the macula are associated with decreased visual acuity or central field defects. The characteristic ophthalmological appearance includes perivascular fluffy yellow-white retinal infiltrates, and focal necrotizing retinitis with or without intraretinal haemorrhage. There is very little inflammation of the vitreous. Blood vessels near the lesions might be sheathed. The lesions might have a granular appearance. In the absence of HAART or specific anti-CMV therapy, retinitis progresses and causes a characteristic brushfire pattern, usually within 10-21 days after presentation. A granular, white leading edge forms, eventually resulting in an atrophic and gliotic scar leading to blindness.

CMV colitis is the second most common manifestation, and occurs in 5-10% of patients with CMV infection. The most frequent clinical manifestations are fever, weight loss, anorexia, abdominal pain, diarrhoea and malaise. Extensive mucosal haemorrhage and perforation can cause life-threatening complications.

CMV oesophagitis occurs in less than 5% and causes fever, odynophagia, nausea and mid-epigastric or retrosternal discomfort. Pneumonitis is uncommon, but can cause shortness of breath, dyspnoea on exertion, a nonproductive cough and hypoxaemia.

CMV neurological disease causes dementia, ventriculoencephalitis, or ascending polyradiculomyelopathy. Patients with dementia typically have lethargy, confusion and fever.The condition might mimic HIV dementia.

DIAGNOSIS

CMV viraemia can be detected by PCR, antigen assays or blood culture. A negative IgG antibody suggests that CMV is unlikely to have caused disease. Patients with advanced immunosuppression might serorevert from being antibody-positive to -negative.

The diagnosis of CMV retinitis is based on characteristic retinal changes in the fundus. CMV colitis is recognized by mucosal ulcerations on endoscopic examination and colonoscopic or rectal biopsy. Histopathology demonstrates characteristic intranuclear and intracytoplasmic inclusions. The diagnosis of CMV oesophagitis is established by the presence of extensive large, shallow ulcers in the distal oesophagus. Biopsy shows intranuclear inclusion bodies in the endothelial cells with an inflammatory reaction at the edge of the ulcer. Culturing CMV from a biopsy or cells brushed from the colon or the oesophagus is not sufficient to establish the diagnosis.

The diagnosis of CMV pneumonitis should be made with X-ray evidence of pulmonary interstitial infiltrates. CMV inclusion bodies can be identified in the lung tissue.

CMV neurological disease is diagnosed on the basis of the clinical syndrome and the presence of CMV in the CSF or brain tissue. The use of PCR enhances the detection of CMV. The CSF generally demonstrates lymphocytic pleocytosis; there may be a mixture of neutrophils and lymphocytes. The glucose levels may be low-to-normal, and protein levels normal-to-high. Periventricular enhancement on CT or MRI images helps to distinguish CMV ventriculoencephalitis from HIV-1-related neurological disease.

LABORATORY DIAGNOSIS

The diagnosis of CMV infection requires laboratory confirmation and cannot be made on clinical grounds alone. CMV antigen detection can be done using commercially available kits. Virus isolation and PCR can be done by State/National Laboratories.

The presence of CMV IgM antibody is useful but not a reliable indicator of an acute infection. IgM antibodies may not be present during an active infection (false-negative) or may persist for such a long time that the finding may not be diagnostic (false-positive).

Polymerase chain reaction (PCR): PCR using primers from a part of a genome coding for immediate early antigen has been used but this method is oversensitive. RT-PCR for CMV RNA or quantitative PCR to determine the CMV load is more useful in detecting active infection or monitoring antiviral therapy.

TREATMENT

Treatment suppresses the infection and prevents relapse. It cannot reverse damage that has already occurred. Treatment for CMV retinitis can be given intravenously, orally, or directly into the eye(s). It consists of two phases: induction therapy and maintenance therapy. Induction therapy usually takes two or three weeks.

Maintenance therapy is intended to prevent the virus from causing a relapse. This may be discontinued once the CD4 count increases to more than 200 cells/mm^3 for at least 6 months following HAART. The treatment of choice is ganciclovir 5 mg/kg twice daily IV (induction) followed by capsules (maintenance), and can treat all forms of CMV disease. IV ganciclovir is given twice daily for two to three weeks and then IV once daily 5-7 days a week. Oral treatment is given as 1000 mg capsules three times daily.

Intravenous foscarnet can be used to treat CMV retinitis and all other forms of CMV disease. It is given 2-3 times daily for two to three weeks and then once a day.

Intravenous cidofovir with probenecid (to help prevent kidney damage) is given once a week for two weeks. It has been studied only in CMV retinitis but might be effective in other forms of the disease.

Valganciclovir may be given orally as two 450 mg tablets twice a day for three weeks, followed by two 450 mg tablets once a day. It is the only treatment for CMV that can be given orally. It has been shown to be as effective as IV ganciclovir for the treatment of CMV retinitis. It has many of the side-effects of IV ganciclovir.

Ganciclovir implants have been used in the past, although they have a high incidence of recurrence and retinal detachment.

OTHER DISORDERS

HIV Associated Neurocognitive Disorders (HAND) can occur when HIV enters the nervous system and impacts the health of nerve cells. This, in turn, can impair the activity of nerves involved in:
- Attention
- Memory
- Language
- Problem solving
- Decision making
- Confusion
- Forgetfulness
- Behavioral changes

- Headaches
- Gradual weakening and loss of feeling in the arms and legs
- Problems with cognition or movement
- Pain due to nerve damage

TYPES OF HIV ASSOCIATED NEUROCOGNITIVE DISORDERS (HAND)

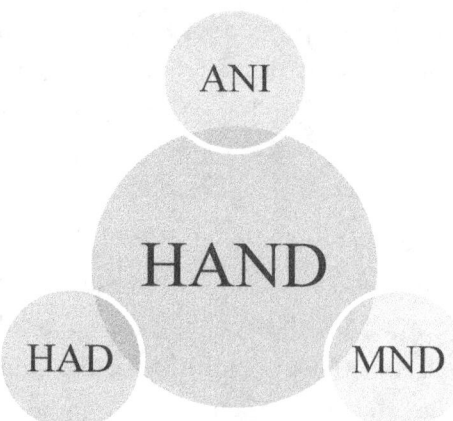

- **Asymptomatic Neurocognitive Impairment (ANI)** is diagnosed if testing shows HIV-associated impairment in cognitive function, but everyday functioning is not affected.
- **Mild Neurocognitive Disorder (MND)** is diagnosed if testing shows HIV-associated impairment in cognitive function, and mild interference in everyday functioning.
- **HIV-associated Dementia (HAD)** is diagnosed if testing shows marked impairment in cognitive function, especially in learning of new information, information processing, and attention or concentration. This impairment significantly limits your ability to function day-to-day at work, home, and during social activities.

DIAGNOSIS

Many factors can contribute to the same types of symptoms as HAND, making diagnosis a complex and challenging task. Depression, other psychiatric disturbances, reactions to medication, and nutritional deficiencies can all lead to similar symptoms. Infections common among people with advanced HIV can also lead to these symptoms, although typically only among those not on cART (e.g. toxoplasmosis, lymphoma, progressive multifocal leukoencephalopathy (PML) and cryptococcal meningitis).

An accurate diagnosis of HAND, therefore, requires a comprehensive examination that generally includes a mental status test, a brain scan, and sometimes lab tests on the cerebrospinal fluid (the fluid that bathes the brain and spinal cord), which are obtained through a procedure known as a spinal tap or lumbar puncture. A mental status exam can help identify whether a person is suffering from memory loss, difficulties with concentration and other thinking processes, mood swings, and other symptoms. The best diagnosis requires a third party (e.g. friend, partner, or other family member) corroborate the behavior/memory changes.

Because no single test definitively answers the question of whether someone has HAND, the final diagnosis is made by weighing all the evidence together. Time and repeated measures are helpful in confirming a diagnosis.

TREATMENT

Although there is no cure for HAND, the single most important treatment is adherence to antiretroviral therapy to maintain a suppressed viral load in the blood. The specific medicines that make up the cART regimen appear to be less important than just being on a regimen. In rare cases, doctors may have to consider how well these medicines get into the central nervous system and there are studies underway to see if some medications may help symptoms better than others. These new findings, however, should not cloud our understanding that suppression of plasma virus to undetectable or unquantifiable levels in blood appears to be most critical.

Knowing the diagnosis is also sometimes therapeutic, as there is stigma and stress related to these symptoms and how they affect daily activities. These can be addressed with proper diagnosis. Knowing that the illness exists may also prompt compensatory approaches and, ultimately, decrease stress and anxiety.

In addition to treating HAND itself, it is important to find ways to treat the secondary symptoms when possible. Anti-depressants, anti-psychotics, and anti-anxiety drugs can help relieve some of the mental distress people with HAND may experience. However, some of these medications may cause complications when taken along with antiretroviral therapy or other drugs; caution is needed in choosing the best approach. Consultation with an HIV-knowledgeable doctor is recommended.

It is also important that patients engage in their own care to prevent factors that can contribute to cognitive symptoms. This includes aggressive treatment of depression, good health care maintenance to address common comorbidities (e.g. hypertension, lipid abnormalities, liver impairment), avoiding non-prescription drugs and excessive alcohol, working with care providers to assure that the medications taken are all required, and exercise. There is growing evidence that physical exercise is important. Optimally, this can be done while engaging in other activities, since social integration and activities may also be helpful. Keeping engaged with enjoyable activites likely translates into benefits.

HOW ARE HAND DIAGNOSED AND TREATED?

Experienced neurologists can diagnose HAND after carefully ruling out other possible causes of the symptoms. They may conduct a thorough neurological exam and history, brain MRI scan, and sometimes lumbar puncture to evaluate the cerebrospinal fluid. Neuropsychological testing can add useful information about the nature and severity of HAND. Talk to your doctor if you think you have symptoms of HAND.

REFERENCES

American Academy of Neurology AIDS Task Force (1991) Nomen-clature and research case definitions for neurological manifes-tations of human immunodeficiency virus type-1 (HIV-1) infection. American Academy of Neurology, St. Paul

Antinori A, Arendt G, Becker JT, Brew BJ, Byrd DA, Cherner M, Clifford DB, Cinque P, Epstein LG, Goodkin K, Gisslen M, Grant I, Heaton RK, Joseph J, Marder K, Marra CM, McArthur JC, Nunn M, Price RW, Pulliam L, Robertson KR, Sacktor N, Valcour V, WojnaVE (2007) Updated research nosology for HIV-associated neuro-cognitive disorders. Neurology

Beck AT, Brown GK, Steer RA (1996) Beck depression inventory, 2nd edition manual. The Psychological Corporation, San Antonio

Centers for Disease Control and Prevention (2000) HIV surveillance report, 2000, vol 12. Centers for Disease Control and Prevention, Atlanta

Dore GJ, McDonald A, Li Y, Kaldor JM, Brew BJ (2003) Marked improvement in survival following AIDS dementia complex in the era of highly active antiretroviral therapy. AIDS

Family Caregiver Alliance (2015), HIV-associated Neurocognitive Disorder (HAND) [Reserved from; https://www.caregiver.org/hiv-associated-neurocognitive-disorder-hand]

Morgello S, Singer EJ, Grant I, Heaton RK (2004) Interrater reliability of clinical ratings and neurocognitive diagnoses in HIV. J Clin Exp Neuropsychol

Naco (2007) Guidelines for Prevention and Management of Common Opportunistic Infection/Malignancies among HIV-Infected Adults and Adolescent; Ministry of Health and Family Welfare, Government of India, New Delhi

The National Institute of Mental Health (NIMH) (2015); HIV Associated Neurocognitive Disorders [Reserved from: http://www.nimh.nih.gov/health/topics/hiv-aids/hiv-associated-neurocognitive-disorders.shtml]

White DA, Heaton RK, Monsch AU (1995) Neuropsychological studies of asymptomatic human immunodeficiency virus-type-1 infected individuals. J Int Neuropsychol Soc 1

Woods SP, Rippeth JD, Frol AB, Levy JK, Ryan E, Soukup VM, Hinkin CH, Lazzaretto D, Cherner M, Marcotte TD, Gelman BB,

World Health Organization (1997) Composite international diagnostic interview, version 2.1. WHO, Geneva

Image Credit

Figure 1; MR angiography of large vessel stenosis after cryptococcal meningitis by Arnold Kang, David Haynor

Figure 2, (Left) Axial T2-Weighted image shows a left temporal lobe mass with surrounding edema (black arrows) other small lesions are seen in right parietal lobe (white arrows) by Pinterest

Figure 3, (Right) Axial contrast T1-weighted image shows nodular and irregular ring enhancement (black arrows), small enhancing lesions are seen in bilateral cerebral hemispheres (white arrows) by Pinterest

Figure 4, Cytomegalovirus Infection by Flickr

Impact of Corporate Social Responsibility for Deal and Preventing HIV/AIDS at Working Place

Mr. Parmanand Barodiya[5], Dr. Abdesh Singh Kushwah[6], Miss. Anita Singh Chauhan[7]

ABSTRACT

HIV/AIDS had developed into a major threat that had a devastating effect on human resources and economies throughout the world. The corporate sector had woken up to this threat and was engaged in various HIV/AIDS related corporate social responsibility (CSR) efforts to help the victims and spread awareness. Workplace policies aim to manage sensitive issues, such as confidentiality of medical information and continuation of employment for HIV- positive staff, and assure that all testing and counseling services are performed on a voluntary rather than mandatory basis. Many prominent companies have already formalized their policies and programmes related to HIV/AIDS in the workplace.

Keywords: HIV, AIDS, Workplace, Management, CSR, (HRM)

The role of the private sector is critical if efforts to fight AIDS in India are to be effective and sustainable. Business possesses valuable resources that can easily and cost-effectively be utilized, such as financial resources, management and marketing skills, meeting space and fora, and access to workers, consumers and communities. This brochure describes how companies can immediately protect their economic, social and human resource interests by providing healthy

---

[5] Research Scholar of Commerce Dept. Madhav Mahavidyalaya, Gwalior (MP), India

[6] Asst. Prof. of Commerce & Management Dept. Preston College, Gwalior (MP), India

[7] Management Department VISM College, Gwalior (MP), India

occupational settings that acknowledge the potential impact of HIV/AIDS in the workplace.

Many companies nowadays have health care plans for ill employees, formal policies and educational efforts, particularly in regard to HIV, are often neglected. Developing such policies and practices should be seen as an investment, protecting a core business asset - the talent pool. Overall, the response of business in Asia to HIV/AIDS needs to be further advanced. While infection rates in Asia are rising rapidly, implementation of HIV/AIDS workplace management policies and programmes is lagging, creating a serious threat to corporate resources. If business does not respond with strong prevention efforts now, they can expect much greater challenges for care and treatment in the coming years. The hesitancy of many companies to invest in HIV/AIDS prevention may be due to a lack of data on the macro-economic impact of HIV, as well as a perceived lack of support mechanisms and technical assistance for business engaged in HIV prevention activities. It may also reflect a perception that HIV/AIDS is self-inflicted and therefore not a company or corporate responsibility.

OBJECTIVE:

- ✓ To Study of HIV/AIDS & Corporate social responsibility.
- ✓ To know Symptoms of HIV/AIDS infection.
- ✓ To know how can deal with HIV/AIDS at working place.
- ✓ To know how can prevent HIV/AIDS at working place.

RESEARCH METHODOLOGY:

The researchers have adopted descriptive methodology for this study Research has been placed on secondary data sources such as books, journals, newspapers and online database.

Corporate Social Responsibility:

There is little consensus on the definition of Corporate Social Responsibility; however, most definitions describe CSR as a concept whereby companies integrate social and environmental concerns in their business operations and in their interactions with their stakeholders on a voluntary basis. The "Karmayog CSR Study and Ratings of Indian Companies" states that CSR is about two aspects:

- ✓ "The steps taken by the company to neutralize, minimize, or offset the negative effects caused by its processes and product-usage".
- ✓ "The further positive steps a company takes using its resources, core competence, skills, location, and funds for the benefit of people and environment" (Karmayog, 2009).

The World Business Council for Sustainable Development defines CSR as "the continuing commitment by business to behave ethically and contribute to economic development while improving the quality of life of the workforce and their families as well as of the local community and society at large" (Collage Article 13, 2007).

What is HIV?

"HIV" stands for Human Immunodeficiency Virus. To understand what that means, let's break it down:

- ✓ H – Human – This particular virus can only infect human beings.
- ✓ I – Immunodeficiency – HIV weakens your immune system by destroying important cells that fight disease and infection. A "deficient" immune system can't protect you.
- ✓ V – Virus – A virus can only reproduce itself by taking over a cell in the body of its host.

HIV is a lot like other viruses, including those that cause the "flu" or the common cold. But there is an important difference – over time, your immune system can clear most viruses out of your body. That isn't the case with HIV – the human immune system can't seem to get rid of it. That means that once you have HIV, you have it for life.

What is AIDS?

"AIDS" stands for Acquired Immunodeficiency Syndrome. To understand what that means, let's break it down:

- ✓ A – Acquired – AIDS is not something you inherit from your parents. You acquire AIDS after birth.
- ✓ I – Immuno – Your body's immune system includes all the organs and cells that work to fight off infection or disease.
- ✓ D – Deficiency – You get AIDS when your immune system is "deficient," or isn't working the way it should.
- ✓ S – Syndrome – A syndrome is a collection of symptoms and signs of disease. AIDS is a syndrome, rather than a single disease, because it is a complex illness with a wide range of complications and symptoms.

As noted above, AIDS is the final stage of HIV infection, and not everyone who has HIV advances to this stage. People at this stage of HIV disease have badly damaged immune systems, which put them at risk for opportunistic infections (OIs). You are considered to have progressed to AIDS if you have one or more specific OIs, certain cancers, or a very low number of CD4 cells. If you have AIDS, you will need medical intervention and treatment to prevent death.

Symptoms of HIV/AIDS infection:

Many people with HIV/AIDS have no symptoms for several years. Others may develop symptoms similar to flu, usually two to six weeks after catching the virus. The symptoms can last up to four weeks. Symptoms of early HIV/AIDS infection May include

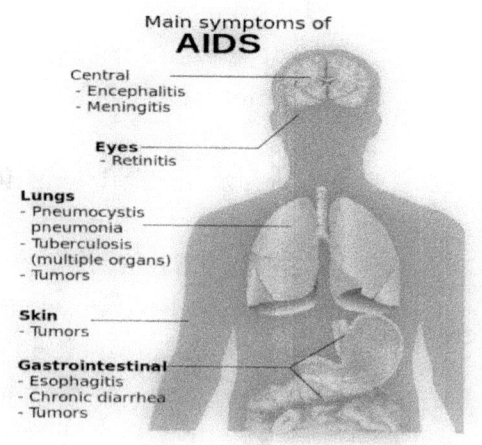

Main symptoms of
AIDS

Central
- Encephalitis
- Meningitis

Eyes
- Retinitis

Lungs
- Pneumocystis pneumonia
- Tuberculosis (multiple organs)
- Tumors

Skin
- Tumors

Gastrointestinal
- Esophagitis
- Chronic diarrhea
- Tumors

- ✓ Fever
- ✓ Chills
- ✓ Joint pain
- ✓ Muscle ache
- ✓ Sore throat
- ✓ Sweats (particularly at night)
- ✓ Enlarged glands
- ✓ A red rash
- ✓ Tiredness
- ✓ Weakness
- ✓ Weight loss

HIV/AIDS & Corporate Social Responsibility:

Corporate Social Responsibility as "achieving commercial success in ways that honors ethical values and respect people, communities and natural environment". We also say that CSR means addressing the legal, ethical, commercial and other expectations society has for business and making decisions that fairly balance the claims of the key stakeholders. In its simplest terms it is "What you do, how you do it, and when and what you say". Underlining the economic cost of the epidemic, the then Chairman of the National Business Alliance on HIV/AIDS (NBA) Hadi S. Topobroto said at the opening ceremony of the Asia-Pacific HIV/AIDS Private Sector Mobilization in Indonesia, a country where 15 percent of the population is living with HIV/AIDS would suffer a one percent decrease in GDP per year. Therefore, employers and company owners have the responsibility to protect their workers from the spread of the HIV/AIDS epidemic". Therefore the corporate social responsibility efforts against HIV/AIDS are on the rise.

Dealing with HIV/AIDS in the working place:

The human immunodeficiency virus (HIV), which causes acquired immunodeficiency syndrome (AIDS), has led to great concern in the workplace in recent years. The majority of people infected with HIV/AIDS are between the ages of 20 to 45 and are employed, many by small and mid-sized businesses. This raises questions regarding the measures an employer must take to accommodate these employees. Despite the ramifications of HIV/AIDS in the workplace, few companies have an established policy to guide their response to this issue.

- **HIV Testing as a Condition of Employment-** Several states prohibit HIV/AIDS testing as a condition of employment, while others permit HIV/AIDS testing when the employer can show a legitimate reason for doing so. To establish a legitimate reason, there must be some connection between HIV/AIDS and job performance or safety. This connection may exist when the job involves a risk of transmitting the disease. An employer, who tests for HIV/AIDS without a legitimate reason, or who does so merely because of suspicion that the employee is a homosexual or drug user, may be liable for an invasion-of-privacy claim by the job applicant.

- **Rights of Co-Workers-** Certain federal laws allow employees to discontinue working when they have a reasonable belief that their working conditions are unsafe. Given the consensus in the medical field that HIV/AIDS cannot be transmitted through casual contact, it would be difficult for an employee to refuse on these grounds to work with an HIV/AIDS infected co-worker. The reasonableness of the employee's demand may depend on how the employer has educated employees about HIV/AIDS. If the employees have been taught that HIV/AIDS cannot be transmitted through casual contact, their refusal to work may be found to be "unreasonable" and they could be discharged.

- **Accommodations for HIV/AIDS Employees-** Federal legislation not only prohibits discrimination against handicapped persons, but also requires employers to make reasonable efforts to accommodate handicapped applicants and employees where obstacles exist that would impede their employment opportunities. Insofar as an employee with HIV/AIDS is considered handicapped, an employer must make reasonable accommodations for him or her. In addition, if your company is covered by the Rehabilitation Act and an employee has HIV/AIDS or develops it, you must make reasonable accommodations that permit the employee to continue working in the position. Such accommodations can include leave policies, flexible work schedules, reassignment to vacant positions and part-time employment. The criteria used to determine whether an employer is making reasonable accommodations for an HIV/AIDS-infected employee include the cost of the accommodation, the size of the business and the nature of the employee's work.

- **Guidelines to Consider-** Through advance education and preparation, an employer can avoid many of the problems associated with employees infected with HIV. When dealing with HIV issues, employers should:
  - ✓ adopt an up-to-date HIV/AIDS education program that discussed how HIV is transmitted and explains the company's policies regarding employees with HIV/AIDS;
  - ✓ treat HIV/AIDS infected employees in the same manner as other employees suffering from disabilities or illnesses are treated under company health plans and policies;
  - ✓ allow HIV/AIDS-infected employees to continue working as long as they are able to perform their jobs satisfactorily and their continued employment does not pose a safety threat to themselves, other employees, or customers;
  - ✓ make reasonable efforts to accommodate HIV/AIDS-infected employees by providing them with flexible work hours and assignments; and
  - ✓ Protect all information regarding an HIV/AIDS-infected employee's condition.

There is a broad range of legal issues that companies must consider when formulating their practices and responses toward HIV/AIDS. By educating your employees, you may be able to reduce the work disruption, legal implications, financial implications and other effects that HIV/AIDS can have on your business. Given the complexity and changing nature of HIV/AIDS, an employer should always examine the laws applicable in its jurisdiction and consult an attorney when handling HIV/AIDS issues in the workplace.

Workplace programmers:

- **HIV/AIDS policy development-** A policy structures all efforts related to workplace prevention of HIV/AIDS and mitigation of its Effects. The policy not only formalizes the company's commitment to manage HIV/AIDS, but also shares the responsibilities for upholding the policy with company employees. Shell Philippines decided to implement an HIV/AIDS policy after an assessment was made of the costs Related to prevention. Management concluded that a formalized HIV/AIDS policy would result in greater budget efficiencies compared to non-intervention.

- **Executive briefing -** The executive briefing targets senior management, such as the CEO, Executive Director and Board of Advisors. This 1-2 hour curriculum aims to brief decision making management on the macro- and microeconomic impact of HIV/AIDS and basic issues of workplace intervention, prevention and care and support, such as education, policy development, legal issues and assistance to HIV-positive employees.

- **Human resource management (HRM) training-** HRM training provides guidance for human resource managers and supervisors in complying with policy regulations, managing potential workplace conflict and accommodating the needs of HIV-positive employees. This curriculum is usually provided in one day, but its duration can be tailored to the size of the company.

- **Staff training-** Training of employees is the backbone of any workplace prevention programme. This 3-4 hour curriculum

46

aims to build staff knowledge and capacity to analyze personal risk behavior and prevent HIV transmission. An increased understanding of HIV/AIDS will further help staff to feel comfortable working together with HIV-positive co-workers.

- **Workplace care and support measures-** Provision of reasonable care and support services is essential to enable HIV-positive employees to continue working as long as possible and fulfill their expected job responsibilities. Accommodating the needs of both management and HIV-positive staff is a process of problem solving balanced by guidelines as described in the HIV/AIDS policy. Rohm Apollo Electronics in Thailand financially supports HIV-positive employees who become ill and allows them to change to other positions in the company to facilitate their ability to continue working for as long as possible. There exists a wide variety of possible care and support provisions.

CSR for the prevention of HIV/AIDS:

The role of Corporate Social Responsibility and active involvement of the private sector in the response to HIV/AIDS epidemic has been gaining momentum in the region during the last few years as Several Indian companies, including Larsen & Toubro, Tata Tea Limited, Aditya Birla Group, Apollo Tyres, Modicare Foundation, SAIL and Bajaj Auto, have also launched preventive efforts. There are many encouraging examples of CSR, Pubic-Private partnerships and the private and corporate sectors demonstrating active roles in prevention, care and support activities. Promoting CSR in HIV/AIDS prevention, care and support initiatives in the Asia Pacific region is one of the objectives of the advocacy and communication efforts of the UNDP Regional HIV and Development Programme. In partnership with other stakeholders and private and corporate sectors, the idea is to create a regional platform for fostering CSR in HIV/AIDS.

SAIL (The Steel Authority of India Limited) has initiated a prevention and control of HIV/AIDS programme titled "SAIL AIDS Control Programme" (SACP) in association with the National AIDS Control Organization (NACO). As part of inter-sectoral collaboration, SAIL has initiated a multi-pronged programme for implementing the policies and guidelines of NACO in its plants/units townships. SAIL's major initiatives include:

✓ School AIDS Education Programme;
✓ Family Health Awareness Campaign;
✓ Safe Blood and Blood Products;
✓ Voluntary Counselling and Testing Centre (VCTC)
✓ World AIDS Day Celebrations;
✓ Exhibition and displays
✓ Counseling and guidance with the help of NGOs.
✓ Establishing ART Centres.

CONCLUSION:

Many companies play a crucial role in HIV/AIDS prevention and support efforts. Mobilization of corporate resources, such as management and marketing expertise, human resources, and funds is especially effective in developing markets where public resources are limited. The rationale for business to engage in workplace programmes to protect their employees from HIV/AIDS is clear. HIV/AIDS impacts on many social and economic issues, such as occupational health and safety, staff morale, human rights and the availability of a productive and well-educated workforce.

REFERENCE:

Anupam Sharma, Corporate Social Responsibility: Driving Forces and Challenges, International Journal of Business Research and Development ISSN 1929- 0977 | Vol. 2 No. 1, pp. 18-27 (2013)

Business taking action to manage HIV/AIDS. A selection of business practices responding to HIV/AIDS in- and outside the Asian workplace.

Dr.S.Naya, HIV /AIDS and Corporate Social Responsibility: A Global Challenge, International Journal of Research In Social Sciences, Jan. 2015. Vol. 4, No.9

Vikramjit kaur, Corporate Social Responsibility (CSR): Overview of Indian Corporate,International Journal of Management and Social Science s Research (IJMSSR),Volume 1, No. 3, December 2012

Webs:

en.wikipedia.org/wiki/HIV/AIDS

http://www.entrepreneurship.org/resource-center/dealing-with-hivaids-in-the-workplace.aspx

http://www.hks.harvard.edu/m-rcbg/CSRI/publications/WorkingPaper_8_nelson.pdf

http://www.medicalnewstoday.com/articles/17131.php#signs_and_symptoms

www.aids.gov/hiv-aids-basics/hiv-aids-101/what-is-hiv-aids/

Psychological Well-Being in HIV/AIDS Positive and Negative

Prof. Anjali Srivastava[8], Mohammad Amin Wani[9]

ABSTRACT

This research paper is an attempt to study the level of psychological Well-being in HIV/AIDS patients and normal persons .This study is based on sample of 100 subjects 50 HIV/AIDS patients (25 males and 25 females) and 50 subjects were normal person's (25 males and 25 females). The psychological well-being of HIV/AIDS positive and negative persons were measured by psychological Well-being scale (PWBS) (HINDI) adopted by S. N. Rai & Deepika Gupta Department of Psychology Chaudhary Charan Singh University Meerut. Three independent variables were studied i.e. gender, normality and HIV/AIDS. Mean, S.D and t-test were applied for data analysis. The results reveal that the all three independent variables i.e. gender, normality and HIV/AIDS are found significant at .01 level of confidence. This study shows that there is significant difference between the Psychological Well-being of HIV/AIDS patients and normal's. Significant difference between six areas of psychological Well-being (Self-acceptance, personal growth, purpose in life, environmental mastery, autonomy, positive relations with others) among HIV/AIDS patients and normal's were found. Also significant difference was found between male and female HIV/AIDS patients.

Keywords: Psychological well-being, HIV/AIDS, Normality, Gender

AIDS (Acquired immunodeficiency syndrome) is a sexually transmitted infection caused by a HIV (Human immunodeficiency virus) that destroys the body's immune system. This virus mainly infects white blood cells called CD4 cells or T helper cells and

---

[8] Professor and Head, Department of Psychology, APS University Campus, Rewa, M.P

[9] Student, M.Phil, Psychology, APS University campus, Rewa, M.P

monocytes; these cells have important functions in the immune system they make the proteins in the body that fight germs and infections to protect the body. When HIV enters the body, it attacks the CD4 cells and minimizes their functions. Which results the immune system weakened, and the body is less able to fight infection. If the number of healthy cells in the body continues to decline, HIV status will changes from HIV positive to AIDS. AIDS occurs when the number of CD4 cells in the body drops below200 cells/μl. By this the body can get HIV-related infections, called opportunistic infections.

HIV is found in the body fluids of an infected person via semen and vaginal fluids, blood and breast milk. These fluids can be passed from one to another variety of ways, including having unprotected sex (oral, vaginal, or anal) or sharing infected needles. HIV can also be passed from mother to child during childbirth or through breast-feeding. Both the virus and the disease are often referred to together as HIV/AIDS.

Acquired Immune Deficiency Syndrome (AIDS) was first clinically observed in the United States in 1981. The initial cases were injecting drug users and homosexual men with no known cause of impaired immunity. Up to 1981 there was no official name of this disease but in general press the term "GRID" was used which stands gay related immune deficiency. The term AIDS was firstly introduced at a meeting in July 1982. In September 1982 the Centers for Disease Control and Prevention (CDC) started referring to the disease as Acquired Immune Deficiency Syndrome (AIDS). In India in 1986 the first known case of HIV was diagnosed by Suniti Solmon amongst female sex workers in Chennai.

Psychosocial aspects of people living with HIV/AIDS

People living with HIV/AIDS are in fear, grief, hopelessness, helplessness syndrome, guilt, anxiety disorder, depression, denial, anger, aggression and suicide attempts

Psychological Well-being

The term Psychological Well-being is defined as people's evaluations of their own lives. Such evaluations can be both cognitive judgments, such as life satisfaction, and there emotional responses to events, such as feeling positive emotions. It is a wide concept includes different aspects of everyday experience. How people think, feel, behave, take decisions etc.

Levi (1987) defined psychological Well-being as "a dynamic state characterized by reasonable amount of harmony between individual's abilities, needs, and expectations, and environmental demands and opportunities".

According to Ryff (1989) the concept of psychological or emotional Well-being was originally construe as a challenge in overcoming the hedonistic concept of Well-being in psychology, and with the aspiration of making a distinction between the hedonistic state of comfort and eudemonic process of growth and development by which happiness, and finally also pleasure, is achieved.

Romy *et al.* (2014) investigated pain in people living with HIV/AIDS. Results revealed that prevalence of pain ranged from a point prevalence of 54% to 83% using a three-month recall period. The reported pain was of moderate-to-severe intensity, and pain was reported in one to two and a half different anatomical sites.

Asante (2012) conducted a study on social support and the psychological wellbeing of people living with HIV/AIDS. Results revealed that social support was negative associated with depression and anxiety, older patients experienced higher level of stress than their younger counterparts.

Rajeev et al. (2012) *examined the impact of HIV/AIDS on quality of life of people living with HIV/AIDS. Results revealed the quality of* *life scores for all domains were intermediate in people living with HIV/AIDS. There was a significant difference in quality of life of people living with HIV/AIDS who was on ART and not on ART in some domains.*

Vanisri *et al.* **(2012)** investigated the death anxiety and Psychological well-being of HIV +ve patients and HIV TB co-infected patients. The found significant difference between male and female HIV +ve patients and HIV TB co-infected patients in death anxiety and psychological well-being.

Gafar et al. (2010) conducted a study on HIV/AIDS and well-being. The result revels that the prevalence of HIV/AIDS has little or no significant impact on well-being in the sub-regions.

Basavaraj *et al.* **(2010)** examined the quality of life in HIV/AIDS. They found that the relevance and complexity of physical, psychological, and social factors as determinants of health-related quality of life in HIV-infected persons.

Sun et al. (2007) examined Psychological status, coping, and social support of people living with HIV/AIDS in central China. Results indicated the HIV/AIDS patients have high levels of psychological distress and their coping style was confrontation.

Sengendo and Nambi (1997) investigated the psychological effect of orphan hood on HIV/AIDS. They found HIV/AIDS orphans had significantly higher depression and lower optimism about the future than non-orphans.

Catz et al. (2002) examined the psychological distress among minority and low income women living with HIV. Results revealed greater anxiety depression symptoms were associated with women who reported higher stress, using fewer active coping strategies and perceiving less social support.

Leserman et al. (2000) *investigated the impact of stressful life events, depression, social support, coping, and cortisol on progression to AIDS. Results revealed AIDS was associated with higher cumulative average stressful life events, coping by means of denial and higher serum cortisol as well as with lower cumulative average satisfaction with social support.*

METHODOLOGY

Statement of the problem:-

To study the level of psychological Well-being in HIV/AIDS patients and normal persons

Hypotheses:-

On the basis of the problem selected in this study following hypotheses are formulated:-

1. There would be a significant difference found between the mean scores of psychological Well-being of HIV/AIDS patients and normal persons
2. There would be significant difference found between six areas of psychological Well-being among HIV/AIDS patients and normal's
3. There would be a significant difference found between the male and female HIV/AIDS patients

Variables:-

Independent Variable: - Gender, normality and HIV/AIDS

Dependent Variable: - Psychological well-being

Sample: - In the present study 100 subjects were selected among which 50 subjects were HIV/AIDS patients (25 males and 25 females) and 50 subjects were normal person's (25 males and 25 females)

Measuring tool:-

In the present study the Psychological Well-being scale (PWBS) (HINDI) adopted by S.N.Rai & Deepika Gupta Department of Psychology C.C.S University Meerut was used. The scale consists 54 items among 28 items are negative and 26 items are positive. The inventory consists of a serious of statements reflecting the six areas of psychological well being Autonomy, environmental mastery, personal growth, positive relations with others, purpose in life, and self acceptance. Respondent's rate statement on a scale of 1 to 6 with 1 indicates strong disagreement and 6 indicates strong agreements.

Positive items are scored as 1, 2, 3,4,5,6 and negative items are scores in reverse form therefore 6, 5, 4,3,2,1 respectively.

The reliability of the scale was checked by test-retest method and was found .77 and the validity was found .75.

RESULTS:-

The main purpose of the present study was to study the level of Psychological Well-being of HIV/AIDS patients and normal persons. The whole data was obtained by using the Psychological well being scale (PWBS) adopted by S.N.Rai & Deepika Gupta Department of Psychology C.C.S University Meerut. The scores were assigned for different responses according to the item. The scores were arranged in tabular form and then t- test was applied to calculate the data. Mean and S.D value of every group was also calculated. Results are given in tables.

Table – 1 Showing means, S.D and t-Value of normal persons and HIV/AIDS patients

Groups	Total scores	N	Mean	σ	df	t-value	Level of significance
Normal persons	10840	50	216.8	13.31	98	20.09**	.01 =2.62
HIV/AIDS Patients	7610	50	152.2	18.43			.05=1.98

*** denotes significant at 0.01 level*

Table-2, Showing means, S.D and t-value of autonomy of normal persons and HIV/AIDS patients

Groups	Total scores	N	Mean	σ	df	t-value	Level of significance
Normal persons	1811	50	36.22	6.85	98	8.29**	.01 =2.62
HIV/AIDS Patients	1277	50	25.54	5.79			.05=1.98

Table-3 Showing means, S.D and t-value of positive growth of normal persons and HIV/AIDS patients

Groups	Total scores	N	Mean	σ	df	t-value	Level of significance
Normal persons	1649	50	32.98	4.28	98	7.99**	.01 =2.62
HIV/AIDS Patients	1260	50	25.2	5.38			.05=1.98

Table-4 Showing means, S.D and t-value of environmental mastery of normal persons and HIV/AIDS patients

Groups	Total scores	N	Mean	σ	df	t-value	Level of significance
Normal persons	1566	50	31.32	3.85	98	5.89**	
							.01 =2.62
HIV/AIDS Patients	1282	50	25.64	5.61			
							.05=1.98

Table-5 Showing means, S.D and t-value of personal growth of normal persons and HIV/AIDS patients

Groups	Total scores	N	Mean	σ	df	t-value	Level of significance
Normal persons	2037	50	40.74	5.02	98	14.68**	
							.01 =2.62
HIV/AIDS Patients	1247	50	24.94	5.71			
							.05=1.98

Table-6 Showing means, S.D and t-value of self acceptance of normal persons and HIV/AIDS patients

Groups	Total scores	N	Mean	σ	df	t-value	Level of significance
Normal persons	1893	50	37.86	4.68	98	10.99**	
							.01 =2.62
HIV/AIDS Patients	1311	50	26.22	5.84			
							.05=1.98

Table-7 Showing means, S.D and t-value of purpose in life *of normal persons and HIV/AIDS patients*

Groups	Total scores	N	Mean	σ	df	t-value	Level of significance
Normal persons	1930	50	38.6	8.99	98	10.1**	.01 =2.62
HIV/AIDS Patients	1233	50	24.66	3.98			.05=1.98

Table-8 Showing means, S.D and t-value of male and female HIV/AIDS patients

Groups	Total scores	N	Mean	σ	df	t-value	Level of significance
Male	4079	25	163.16	16.78	48	5.19**	.01 =2.403
Female	3531	25	141.24	12.71			.05=1.676

*** denotes significant at 0.01 level*

DISCUSSION

The results of the present study suggested that there is significant difference between the psychological Well-being of HIV/AIDS patients and normal persons, as mean scores of HIV/AIDS patients were found 152.2 and normal persons were found 216.2 which are more than mean scores of HIV/AIDS respectively and the t-value is found 20.09 with df 98. Which is more than table value at .01 level of confidence.

Significant difference was found between six areas of psychological Well-being among HIV/AIDS patients and normal's *as the mean scores of all six areas of normal persons are more than mean scores*

58

of HIV/AIDS patients, t-value of all six areas are found more than table value at .01 level of confidence.

Significant difference was found between the male and female HIV/AIDS patients as mean scores of HIV/AIDS male patients were found 163.16 and HIV/AIDS female patients were found141.26 which is less than mean scores of male HIV/AIDS patients and the t-value is found 5.19 with df 48, Which is more than table value at .01 level of confidence.

CONCLUSION

1. *There is a significant difference between the psychological Well-being of HIV/AIDS patients and normal persons.*
2. *There is a significant difference between six areas of psychological Well-being among HIV/AIDS patients and normal's.*
3. *There is a significant difference between psychological well-being of male and female HIV/AIDS patients.*

REFERENCES

Allport, G. (1961). Pattern and growth in personality. New York: Holt, Rinehart, & Winston.

Asante K.O. (2012). Social support and the psychological wellbeing of people living with HIV/AIDS. African Journal of Psychiatry.Vol.15, pages340-345

Basavaraj K., Navya, Rashmi R. (2010). Quality of life in HIV/AIDS. Indian Journal of Sexually Transmitted Diseases and AIDS. Vol. 31, issue 2, pages 75-80.

Catz S. T. et.al (2002). Psychological distress among minority and low income women living with HIV, Behavioral medicine, Vol. 28, issue 2, pages 53-60.

Feldman, Robert S. (1947). Understanding psychology -10th ed. New York, McGraw-Hill, page 373

Gafar T.I., Usman A. R., Abdul W. O.,Olatinwo M. I. and Raji A. B. (2010). HIV/AIDS and well-being in south central and south-east Asia. Pakistan economic and social review. Vol. 48, issue1, pages 85-103

Jane Leserman (2000). Impact of stressful life events, depression, social support, coping, and cortisol on progression to AIDS. The American Journal of Psychiatry Vol. 157, issue 8, pages 1221-1228

Rajeev KH. , Yuvaraj BY. , Nagendra Gowda and Ravikumar. (2012). Impact of HIV/AIDS on quality of life of people living with HIV/AIDS in Chitradurga district, Karnataka. Indian journal of public health. Vol. 56, issue 2, pages 116-121

Romy P., Dan JS. , Jennifer J. (2014). Pain in people living with HIV/AIDS, Journal of the International AIDS Society. Vol. 17, issue 18, page 719

Ryff, C. (1989). Happiness is everything, or is it? Explorations on the meaning of psychological well-being. Journal of Personality and Social Psychology. Vol. 57, pages 1069-1081.

Ryff, C., & Keyes, C. (1995). The structure of psychological well-being revisited. Journal of Personality and Social Psychology. Vol. 69, pages 719-727

Sengendo J., Nambi J. (1997). The psychological effect of orphan hood: a study of orphans in Rakai district. Health Transitions Rev. Vol. 7, pages 105-124.

Sun H., Zhang J., Fu X. (2007). Psychological status, coping and social support of people living with HIV/AIDS in central China. Journal of Public health nursing. Vol 24, issue 2, pages 132-40

Vanisri et.al (2012). Death anxiety and Psychological Well-being of HIV +ve patients and HIV TB co-infected patients, Golden Research Thoughts Volume 2, Issue. 6

Improving Awareness on HIV/AIDS among Adolescents of East Godavari District, Andhra Pradesh

Revathi Sampathirao[10], Ravi Shanker Datti[10]

ABSTRACT

Despite the efforts of the governments on HIV / AIDS awareness it has not been received aptly due to social factors and the stigma attached to the disease. More often the awareness programs are termed under reproductive health education and misunderstood. Most are reluctant to impart awareness due to embarrassment, discomfort with the issues or a lack of knowledge about sexuality. The objective of the present study is to contribute improvement of HIV / AIDS awareness among adolescents of East Godavari district in the context of sexual reproductive rights. A pre-post design has been adopted where in 250 adolescents (mean age 14.08; SD=0.68) from 8 Government High Schools of East Godavari district were assessed prior to and after the intervention. Information on HIV / AIDS education intervention was based on the works of Talking About HIV / AIDS Issues. Participants were assessed using questionnaire on level of awareness on HIV / AIDS issues like pubertal changes, STI/RTI and Human Immunodeficiency Virus / Acquired Immune Deficiency Syndrome (HIV/AIDS). Results show that mean scores in the pubertal changes pre-test was 5.11 and 8.13 in post-test, which increased significantly (t = 35.68, p = 0.001). The mean score in the awareness on STI/RTI pre-test was 3.12 and 6.33 in post-test, which increased significantly (t = 32.53, p = 0.001). The mean score in the awareness on HIV/AIDS pre-test was 4.95 and 7.45 in post-test, which increased significantly (t = 21.79, p = 0.001). The study findings suggest that the intervention improved the participants' awareness on HIV / AIDS issues.

Keywords: HIV/AIDS, Pubertal Changes, STI/RTI and HIV/AIDS

---

[10] Adikavi Nannaya University, Rajahmundry

The adolescents of Andhra Pradesh, like young people everywhere, encounter many challenges to their sexual and reproductive health issues. According to the International Planned Parenthood Federation Framework for Comprehensive Sexuality Education, January 2010 (IPPF), "CSE seeks to equip young people with the knowledge, skills, attitudes and values they need to determine their sexuality- physically and emotionally, individually and in relationships. It views sexuality holistically and within the context of emotional and social development of the youth. It recognizes that information alone is not enough. Young people need to be given the opportunity to acquire essential life skills and develop positive attitudes and values.

Adolescents in Andhra Pradesh are a major group at risk of HIV, sexual transmitted infections (STI), especially with regard to East Godavari and West Godavari districts. Andhra Pradesh (AP) it is considered as one of the country's high HIV/AIDS prevalence states (APSACS, 2009). Adolescent's responses to the risks can have lifelong consequences. Especially the negative physical effects, like poor sexual and HIV / AIDS make them prone to social threats and restrict them to limited educational and employment opportunities. Although recognized by policymakers as a serious public health problem like the NACP III and IV, the health and educational system have not succeeded in responding adequately.

While many adults feel that HIV / AIDS education is important, most are reluctant to take on the responsibility due to embarrassment, discomfort with the issues or a lack of knowledge about sexuality. Compounding to this adolescents being in a crisis stage they face pressures in relation to sex and sexuality from the society. The fear of addressing HIV / AIDS extends to the school as well. This is the place where adolescents spend most of their waking hours, but unfortunately hardly learn anything useful about developing values about sexual health issues.

Though schools have incorporated lessons on reproductive health they are often skipped by the academicians due to underlying discomfort to deal the topics. Another difficulty that adults face in providing HIV / AIDS education is how to impart information and to communicate values without being overly judgemental or forcing opinions. Recent international research conducted by MEMA kwa Vijana (2008) show that to reduce the health risks and avoid the negative outcomes—specifically unintended pregnancy and STIs and HIV— youth not only need accurate information, sexual health education and services, but also a favourable community environment, facilitating youth to make use of the acquired information, tools and services.

Overall objective of this study is to contribute to the improvement of HIV / AIDS awareness among adolescents of East Godavari district in the context of sexual reproductive rights. To provide two day comprehensive information on HIV / AIDS education based workshop. To examine changes in baseline and endline surveys that assess awareness regarding HIV / AIDS issues of adolescents. It is hypothesised that there shall be a significant changes in awareness on SRH issues after the intervention

METHOD

Design
A pre-post research design was conducted where adolescents were evaluated prior to and after the intervention. These scales were administered on day one of the workshop prior to the start of the intervention. The post-intervention assessment was done after completion of the two day workshop. The intervention was carried after obtaining written permission from the school authorities. Variables of the study include Intervention (Independent Variable): The intervention provides 3 day workshop on comprehensive information and skills based on reproductive health education. The activities will provide a framework which will facilitate them to learn about their sexual and reproductive rights. HIV/AIDS Awareness (Dependent Variable): Information acquired to dispel myths; Awareness on references to resources and services available in health and education. Awareness was assessed using questionnaire developed on TARSHI workbook model.

Sample

Stratified Random Sampling technique was considered for the study, with a sample size of 250 adolescents (mean age 14.08; SD=0.68) from 8 Government High Schools of East Godavari district. Of the 250 students 135 (54.4 %) were boys, and 115 (45.6%) were girls. The inclusion criteria were: schools that instruct in Telugu medium; school girls and boys of 14 to 16 years old. The reason for selecting these schools was that the students of it comprise of rural backdrop of East Godavari district.

Intervention

With view of the project goals the intervention program was developed based on the works of TARSHI, Talking About reproductive health Issues, a registered NGO based in New Delhi. TARSHI has developed a highly successful approach using competitive workbook and assessment questionnaire on reproductive health education for adolescent population. The three day HIV / AIDS education program workshop includes interactive learning methods, discussion and reflection, instead of the paradigm of teaching and imposing knowledge and norms.

The activities provide adolescents a framework which will facilitate them to learn about their sexual and HIV / AIDS; acquire information to dispel myths; provide references to resources and services in East Godavari district; obtain skills in communication, negotiation, self development, decision-making; and develop a sense of self, confidence, assertiveness, capacity to take responsibility, seek help and a sense of responsibility. Among the activities are:

• Exercises on getting comfortable
• Harassment and abuse
• Self Esteem and decision making on reproductive rights
• Basic concepts of gender and sexuality
• Prejudice, Stereotypes and Stigma
• The ABC of Anatomy, Physiology, STI/RTI, HIV and AIDS

Tools

HIV / AIDS Questionnaire:

Participants were assessed using a questionnaire on level of awareness on reproductive health issues that include measure on three factors: Pubertal changes, STI/RTI and HIV/AIDS. The questionnaire consists of 10 questions for each factor making it a 30 items questionnaire with yes or no response items. The three factors consisted of items on anatomy and physiology of male/ female reproductive system, physical changes during adolescence, menstrual cycle, contraception, STI/RTI and on HIV/AIDS transmission and preventions. The questionnaire was developed based on the study objectives. The questionnaire was translated into Telugu, the local language by using the back translation technique. The instrument was assessed for the content validity by university faculty of social work department. Scores ranged from 0 to 30 points. The higher the score the more awareness they have about HIV / AIDS issues. As mentioned earlier these scales were administered on day one of the workshop prior to the start of the intervention. The post-intervention assessment was done after completion of the two day workshop.

Statistical Analysis
The study analyzed the data using SPSS to assess the change from pre-test to post-test like paired sample t-test.

RESULTS

Table 1 Profile of the Sample

Variable		N	Mean	S.D.
Age		250	14.08	0.684
Gender	Male	135	14.81	0.693
	Female	115	14.86	0.674

Table 1 shows the profile of the sample with a sample size of 250 adolescents (mean age 14.08; SD=0.68) with age range 14 to 16 years from 8 Government High Schools of East Godavari district. Of the 250 students 135 (54.4 %) were boys, and 115 (45.6%) were girls. The inclusion criteria were: schools that instruct in Telugu medium; school girls and boys of 14 to 16 years old.

Table 2 Pre test Differences among Boys and Girls

Test	Dimensions	Gender	Mean	S.D	t-value
Pre-test	Pubertal Changes	Boys	5.111	.903	.033
		Girls	5.115	.951	
	STI/RTI	Boys	3.140	.534	.626
		Girls	3.097	.550	
	HIV/AIDS	Boys	4.918	1.133	.500
		Girls	4.991	1.145	
	Total Scores	Boys	13.148	1.200	.231
		Girls	13.185	1.346	

From Table 2 we can observe that there are no significant differences were found among boys and girls on HIV / AIDS awareness prior to the intervention. The mean score in the pubertal changes pre-test was 5.111 for boys and 5.115 in girls (t = .033). The mean score on awareness of STI/RTI shows no major changes in pre-test it was 3.140 for boys and 3.097 in girls (t = .626). The mean score in the HIV/AIDS pre-test was 4.918 for boys and 4.991 in girls (t = .500). Similarly no significant differences were found in the overall scores between the groups. Overall performance on the pre test shows that both the groups scored low reflecting their low awareness levels on HIV / AIDS issues. One can also observe that both the groups scored low on STI/RTI issues when compared to pubertal changes and HIV/AIDS.

Table 3 Post test Differences among Boys and Girls

Test	Dimensions	Gender	Mean	S.D	t-value
Post-test	Pubertal Changes	Boys	8.074	.982	.972
		Girls	8.203	1.095	
	STI/RTI	Boys	6.333	1.429	.016
		Girls	6.336	1.497	
	HIV/AIDS	Boys	7.496	1.303	.572
		Girls	7.398	1.379	
	Total Scores	Boys	21.903	3.049	.109
		Girls	21.946	3.170	

From Table 3 we can observe that there are no significant differences found among boys and girls on HIV / AIDS awareness after the two day intervention program. The mean score in the pubertal changes post-test was 8.074 for boys and 8.203 in girls (t = .972). The mean score on awareness of STI/RTI shows no major changes in post-test it was 6.333 for boys and 6.336 in girls (t = .016). The mean score in HIV/AIDS post-test was 7.496 for boys and 7.398 in girls (t = .572). Similarly, no significant differences were found in the overall scores between the groups. Overall performance on the post test shows that both the groups scored better reflecting the effectiveness of the intervention which was targeted to improve their basic levels of understanding on HIV / AIDS issues. One can observe that both the groups improved from their pre test scores in almost all the factors. Both table 2 and table 3 indicate that there are no significant gender differences exist with regard to awareness of HIV / AIDS issues.

Table 4 Changes from Pre-test to Post-test

Dimensions		Pre	Post	t-value
Pubertal	Mean	5.125	7.145	35.780**
Changes	S.D.	.823	1.035	
STI / RTI	Mean	3.122	5.356	32.436**
	S.D.	.541	1.458	
HIV / AIDS	Mean	4.861	6.451	20.856**
	S.D.	1.143	1.336	
Total Scores	Mean	14.165	20.923	36.566**
	S.D.	1.268	3.098	

** $p < .001$

From Table 4 we can observe that there are significant differences found from pre-test assessment to post-test assessment on HIV / AIDS awareness after the two day intervention program. The mean score in the pubertal changes pre-test was 5.11 and 8.13 in post-test, which increased significantly (t = 35.780, p = 0.001). The mean score in the awareness on STI/RTI pre-test was 3.12 and 6.33 in post-test, which increased significantly (t = 32.436, p = 0.001). The mean score in the awareness on HIV/AIDS pre-test was 4.95 and 7.45 in post-test, which increased significantly (t = 20.856, p = 0.001). Overall performance on the post test showed that the adolescents scored high on all dimensions where the mean scores in pre test are 13.165 and 21.923 in post test (t = 36.566, p = 0.001). Though gender differences were not found the overall effectiveness of the intervention was found to be encouraging for the researchers.

DISCUSSION

The findings of the study clearly showed that the two day intervention on HIV / AIDS awareness was effective in imparting awareness among the adolescents of East Godavari district of Andhra Pradesh. The study is unique to the region as life skills education programs on HIV / AIDS issues are carried very rarely, even if they claim, there are no authentic published literature that concerns the needs of adolescents of this region. The present study has introduced a two day intervention program on HIV / AIDS issues awareness to adolescents who are of the age group 14 to 16 years.

The study has revealed some interesting results, one can observe that there are no significant changes on awareness of HIV / AIDS issues between boys and girls. One can assume from the previous literature that there would be gender differences existing due to existing social norms on gender roles and, since girls in general face more problems with regard menarche issues etc., and would receive information from their mothers or significant others (Kotecha, Sangita, Baxi, Mazumdar, Shoba, Ekta and Mansi, 2009). It was observed that there are no such significant differences found. One possible explanation could be that that a significantly large proportion of girls were not aware of menstruation when they first experienced it. Mothers, sisters and friends were found to be the major source of information. Much of this information imparted to a young girl is in the form of restrictions on her movements and behaviour (Anoop, Goyal and Rahul, 2005). One can further explain that both males and females go through the transition from childhood to young adulthood (physical and social). Lack of information and education regarding RH and sexuality is more or less common for both the groups especially adolescents hailing from rural back drop.

It is observed from the study that both the groups has scored very low on STI/RTI issues when compared to other dimensions of the study. Issues in this dimension generally covered sexual infection, including abnormal discharges from genitals, ulcers and sores in the genital region and pelvic infections. Though RTIs can occur both in groups, they are more common in women, because their body structure and functions make it easier for germs to enter. Of concern, however, is that approximately 12–25 percent of all STI cases are among teenage boys (Ramasubban, 1995). Since young and growing children have poor knowledge and lack of awareness about these issues, and parents, who could—or should—be the major source of information and preparation for the transition into adulthood, have largely been uninvolved with educating their children (Gupta, 2003).

Finally the study hypothesised that there would be significant changes on the awareness on HIV / AIDS issues from pre to post test assessment. The findings were in accordance to the research objective. There is significant improvement in all the dimensions under study. As stated by World Health Organisation a complete adolescent HIV / AIDS programme that provide information through didactic education methods like discussions, films, charts, and through participatory methods can influence adolescents behaviour and improve their understanding on HIV / AIDS issues. It has to be noted a program of this nature was never initiated in this region which has high prevalence of HIV/ AIDS. These kind of interventions will not only benefit the direct beneficiaries, but also the communities as a whole, supporting a healthier growing-up of new generations and indirectly benefit the East Godavari region.

CONCLUSION

Certainly the results are encouraging to carry forward such interventions in large scales around these regions as they encourage adolescents in increased utilization of reproductive health services like approaching counsellors, diagnosis and treatment of STIs and pregnancy testing at Government hospitals and area hospitals. This in turn increases the educational and health institutes to be more responsive to adolescent needs. However the present study has certain limitations these include, one the results may not be generalizable to all school adolescents in East Godavari District as only 8 schools were selected. Second this study evaluated the outcomes immediately after the program, it is not certain what the knowledge retention is and for how long it will be retained.

REFERENCES

Andhra Pradesh state annual action plan 2009-10. (2009, February). *Andhra Pradesh State AIDS control Society report to National AIDS Control Organisation.* Retrieved from http://www.apsacs.org/AAP-2009-10.pdf

Anoop, K., Goyal, R.S., and Rahul, B. (2005). Menstrual Practices and Reproductive Problems A Study of Adolescent Girls in Rajasthan. *Journal of Health Management.* Vol. 7 no. 1 91-107. doi: 10.1177/097206340400700103

Comprehensive Sexuality Education. (2010, January). *International Planned Parenthood Federation Framework.* Retrieved from http://www.ippf.org/NR/rdonlyres/ CE7711F7-C0F0-4AF5-A2D5-1E1876C24928/0/Sexuality.pdf

Gupta, S. D. (2003). Adolescent HIV / AIDS in India: Status, Policies, Programs, and Issues. (Contract No. HRN-C-00-00-00006-00). Washington, DC: POLICY Project.

Kotecha, P. V., Sangita Patel, R. K., Baxi, V. S., Mazumdar, S., Ekta, M., and Mansi, D. (2009). HIV / AIDS awareness among rural school going adolescents of Vadodara district. *Indian Journal of Sexually Transmitted Diseases and AIDS.* Jul-Dec; 30(2): 94–99. doi: 10.4103/0253-7184.62765

Long-term Evaluation of the MEMA kwa Vijana (November, 2008). *Adolescent Sexual Health Programme in Rural Mwanza, Tanzania: a Randomised Controlled Trial.* (Technical Briefing Paper: No. 7). Retrieved from http://www.memakwavijana.org/images/stories/Documents/mkv-technical-brief.pdf

Ramasubban, Radhika (1995). Patriarchy and the Risks of STD and HIV Transmission to Women. In Women's Health in India, Oxford: Oxford University Press.

Quality of Life among HIV/AIDS Seroconcordant and Serodiscordant Spouses

Farhat Jahan[11], Professor Akbar Husain[12]

ABSTRACT

HIV/AIDS as we know is an incurable disease. Infection with HIV causes progressive Immunodeficiency resulting in a variety of opportunistic infections which could cause physical and psychological damage and thus decrease PLHIVs (People Living with HIV/AIDS) quality of life. Quality of life is "an individual's perception of his position in life in the context of the culture and value systems in which he lives and in relation to his goals, expectations, standards and concerns" (WHO).

A large number of researches have been done on quality of life among HIV/AIDS patients but quality of life among HIV Seroconcordant and Serodiscordant spouses in North India is not explored. Present study was aimed to investigate quality of life among Seroconcordant and Serodiscordant spouses. The sample consisted of fifty participants (25 Males & 25 Females) of 26 to 60 years of age. Significant differences were not found between the mean scores of comparison groups on dimensions and composite scores of WHOQOL-BREF.

Keywords: *HIV/AIDS, Quality Life, Spouses, Seroconcordant*

Quality of life is a multidimensional approach whose definition and assessment remains controversial (Lessorman, Perkins, & Evans, 2009). Quality of life is conceptualized in terms of "an absence of pain or an ability to function in day to day life. Quality of life as defined by WHO is "individuals' perception of their position in life in the context of the culture and value systems in which they live and

---

[11] Research Scholar, Department of Psychology, A.M.U., Aligarh
[12] Coordinator, UGC-SAP (DRS-1), Department of Psychology, A.M.U. Aligarh

in relation to their goals, expectations, standards and concerns" (WHOQOL-BREF).

The current concept of Quality of life in public health and medicine refers to how the individual's well-being including all physical, psychological, social, spiritual and environmental aspects of the individual's life may be impacted over time by a disease, a disability or a disorder (Dennisor, 2002). Several researchers described Quality of life as a "fighting spirit" associated with longer survival time for individuals (Watchel, Piette, & Mor et al., 1992), (Namir, Fawzy, & Alumbaugh,1992).

Health-related quality of life is an important indicator to assess the impact and quality of health care system. It reflects the patient perspective on various aspects of health, ranging from symptomatic to more complex concepts, such as social functioning or spirituality (Dube & Sattler, 2010). Further as health is generally cited as one of the most important determinants of overall quality of life, it has been suggested that quality of life may be uniquely affected by specific disease process such as AIDS (CDC, 2010), (Rabkin, Remien, Kttoff, & Williams, 1993).

Infection with HIV causes progressive immunodeficiency resulting in a variety of opportunistic infections, which could cause physical and psychological damage and decreased quality of life (Brooks, Kaplan, Holmes, Benson, Pau et al., 2009). Determining the impact on the quality of life in HIV/AIDS patients is important for estimating the burden of the disease. This is true because AIDS has a chronic debilitating course and the long-term adverse side effects of current treatments modalities are uncertain. The social stigma attached with the proclamation of HIV sero-positivity may at times force the individual to change the job or the place of living, putting further stress on the already weak economic situation. This further leads to progressive deterioration of health, low morale, repeated consultation, abstinence from work and low productivity etc. The vicious cycle thus goes on, economic deprivation and social isolation decreases quality of life (Fanning, 1994).

Serodiscordant couple is one in which one spouse is HIV positive and the other spouse is HIV negative. Seroconcordant couple is one in which both the spouses are HIV positive. HIV infected spouses from serodiscordant couples face multiple challenges including the stress of sexual transmission (Attia, Eggerm, Muller, Zwanlen, & Low, 2009). Financial pressures and coping with HIV related stigma all of which may have negative influence on their quality of life (Kalichman, Rompa, Luke, Austin, 2002). On the other hand Seroconcordant spouses face multiple problems such as health related problems of both the partners, danger of death which in turn increases the danger of improper running of family and taking care of children, financial crises, HIV related stigma etc.

Tocco (2009) noted that the popular Islamic hadith, " *For every disease, Allah has given a cure"* is being utilized in Northern Nigeria to assist HIV infected persons to enroll in HIV clinics, consume ARVs, and improve the quality and length of their lives.

Thus, if we look at quality of life, it is positive psychological state which helps individuals in coping with difficult situations and hence, has been assessed in seroconcordant and serodiscordant spouses living with HIV/AIDS.

OBJECTIVES:

- To explore differences between Seroconcordant and Serodiscordant spouses on domains and composite scores on quality of life.
- To examine difference between male and female people living with HIV/AIDS positive on dimensions and composite score on quality of life.

- To examine difference between urban and rural people living with HIV/AIDS on dimensions and composite score on quality of life.

HYPOTHESES:

- There will be no difference between Serodiscordant & Seroconcordant spouses on domains and composite scores on quality of life.
- There will no difference between male and female People living with HIV/AIDS positive on dimensions and composite score on quality of life.
- There will be no difference between urban and rural People living with HIV/AIDS positive on dimensions and composite score on quality of life.

METHOD

Participants

Total sample for the present study comprised of 50 PLHA (People living with HIV/AIDS). Of these, there were 25 male and 25 female Seroconcordant (Positive) and Serodiscordant (Positive and Negative) spouses. They were drawn from ART (Antiretroviral therapy centre), J.N. Medical college, A.M.U., Aligarh. Majority of patients were in the age range of 26-50 years, CD_4 cell count 200-600 cells/ml, WHO clinical stage 1st and 2nd and their monthly income were between 2000-6000 rupees per month.

Tool

WHOQOL-BREF was developed by the WHO QOL group was used in this study (Orley & Kuyken, 1994; Szabo, 1996; WHO QOL group 1994a, 1994b, 1995).The WHOQOL-BREF contains 26 questions. In addition, two items from the overall quality of life and general health facet have been included. The WHOQOL-BREF is based on four domain structure i.e.; Physical health, Psychological, Social relationships and Environment. Cronbach alpha values for each of the four domain scores ranged from .66 (for 3 domains) to .84 (for domain 1). The WHOQOL-BREF has high discriminant validity when compared with WHOQOL-100 in discriminating between the ill and well groups.

Procedure

Seroconcordant (Positive) and Serodiscordant (Positive and Negative) HIV/AIDS spouses were contacted individually and proper rapport was established. Then purpose of the study was explained to each and every participant and participants were assured that their responses will be kept confidential and will be used for research purpose. The data were collected individually through face-to-face interview method.

Data Analysis: t-test was used to analyze the data.

RESULTS AND DISCUSSION

Table 1: Indicating difference between Seroconcordant (Positive) and Serodiscordant (Positive and Negative) Spouses on Domains of Quality of Life

Domains Spouse Status	N	Mean	Std. Deviation	t-value	p
Physical +VE	28	25.46	3.863	-.073	➢ .05
-VE	16	25.56	4.531		
Psychological +VE	28	20.71	3.780	-.209	➢ .05
-VE	16	21.00	4.662		
Social relationships +VE	28	10.07	1.331	-1.658	➢ .o5
-VE	16	10.75	1.291		
Environmental +VE	28	27.46	3.585	-.163	➢ .05
-VE	16	27.69	4.743		

Table: 2 Indicating difference between Seroconcordant (Positive) and Serodiscordant (Positive and Negative) Spouses on Quality of Life

Spouse Status	N	Mean	Std. Deviation	t-value	p
+VE	28	20.93	2.368	-.342	➢ .05
-VE	16	21.25	3.308		

Table 3: Indicating difference between Male and Female HIV Positive on domains of Quality of Life.

Domains Gender	N	Mean	Std. Deviation	t-value	p
Physical					
Male	25	26.16	3.520	1.427	➢ .05
Female	25	24.60	4.183		
Psychological					
Male	25	20.20	4.282	-.167	➢ .05
Female	25	20.40	4.163		
Social relationships					➢ **.05**
Male	25	10.32	1.282	.416	
Female	25	10.16	1.434		
Environmental					
Male	25	27.32	3.705	-.108	➢ **.05**
Female	25	27.44	4.144		

Table 4: Table 1: Indicating difference between Male and Female HIV Positive on Quality of Life.

Gender	N	Mean	Std. Deviation	t-value	p
Male	25	21.00	2.703	.461	➢ .05
Female	25	20.65	2.666		

Table 5: Indicating difference between people with HIV Positive living in Rural and Urban areas on domains of Quality of Life.

Domains Locale	N	Mean	Std. Deviation	t-value	p
Physical Rural	40	24.95	3.909	-1.669	➢ .05
Urban	10	27.10	3.573		
Psychological Rural	40	20.00	3.889	-.847	➢ .05
Urban	10	21.50	5.255		
Social relationships Rural	40	10.15	1.292	-.835	➢ .05
Urban	10	10.60	1.578		
Environmental Rural	40	26.75	3.470	-2.015	< .05
Urban	10	29.90	4.630		

Table 6: Indicating difference between people with HIV Positive living in Rural and Urban areas on Quality of Life.

Locale	N	Mean	Std. Deviation	t-value	p
Rural	40	20.46	2.414	-1.662	➢ .05
Urban	10	22.28	3.231		

Significant differences were not found between Seroconcordant and Serodiscordant spouses, rural and urban PLHA, and male and female PLHA on domains of quality of life and the composite score on quality of life. Urban people living with HIV positive scored significantly higher than rural people living with HIV positive on 'environmental' dimension of quality of life. All hypotheses were accepted.

In the present study it was found that Seroconcordant and Serodiscordant spouses did not differ significantly on any dimension of quality of life. This finding suggests that both type of spouses perceived the same level of physical, psychological, social relationship, and environmental dimensions of quality of life.

Quality of life in HIV Seroconcordant couples may be balanced by their mental attitude and social support. Whereas in the case of Serodiscordant couple the positive spouse may feel that he/she cares for his/her partner because he/she did not transmit HIV to his/her partner. All these things will contribute to their quality of life.

Significant difference was found between people with HIV positive living in rural and urban areas on environment dimension of quality of life. From this finding it can be inferred that both the groups have different lifestyles i.e. they have different timings of sleep and rest, work capacity, financial resources, home environment, opportunity for acquiring new information and skills, leisure time activities, and physical environment.

It is suggested that alone antiretroviral therapy may not necessarily improve quality of life of PLHA cases (Dowdy, 2012). There is a need to provide them psychosocial and spiritual interventions. We should also provide emotional and social support to the seroconcordant and serodiscordant spouses.

CONCLUSION AND IMPLICATIONS:

The motivated patients can improve their situation and health-related quality of life through contentment and developing a sense of meaning in a habitual way. This may be temporary or lasting depending on patients' capacity to improve their quality of life. Spiritual counseling may combine with prayer, meditation, steadfastness and will power.

If we enhance quality of life of PLHA their disease progression will be slow, CD_4 count will increase, adherence will increase and this will in turn improve their overall physical and psychological health.

On the other hand, faith in God and conviction of the higher meaning of life, supported by spiritual values may be essential for their spiritual health and long life. All the practical spiritual principles of thought and activity point to the power within the mind which makes life more meaningful. The inspiring stories of the transforming power of spiritual thought may serve to enlighten and encourage to the HIV people. Adopting healthy lifestyles will improve the quality of life with the highest hopes and expectations.

REFERENCES

Attia, S., Egger, M., Muller, M., Zwahlen, M., & Low, N. (2009). Sexual transmission of HIV according to viral load and antiretroviral therapy: Systematic review and meta-analysis. *AIDS, 23*, 1397–1404.

Brooks, J. T., Kaplan, J. E., Holmes, K. K., Benson, C., Pau, A. et al (2009). HIV associated opportunistic infections-going , going, but not gone: They continued need for prevention and treatment guidelines. *Clinical Infection Disease, 48*, 609-611.

CDC- Health related quality of life (updated 2010 June 3; cited 2011 Feb. 17). National centre for chronic disease. Prevention and health promotion; Available from: http://www.cdc.gov/hrqol.

Dennison, C. R. (2002). The role of patients – reported outcomes in evaluating the quality of Oncology care. *American Journal of Management Care, 8*, S580-586.

Dowdy, D. W. (2012). Quality of life outcomes of Antiretroviral Treatment for HIV/AIDS patients in Vietnam. Johns Hopkins Bloomberg School of Public Health, United States of America.

Dube, M. P., & Sattler, F. R. (2010). Inflammation and Complications of HIV disease. *Journal of Infectious Disease, 201*, 1783-1785.

Fanning, M. (1994).Validation of a QOL instrument for patients with HIV infection. *Health and welfare: Canada* (NHRDP 6606-4334-AIDS).

Kalichman, S. C., Rompa, D., Luke, W., & Austin, J. (2002). HIV transmission risk behaviours among HIV-positive persons in serodiscordant relationships. *International Journal of STD AIDS, 13*, 677–682.

Lessorman, J., Perkins, D. O., & Evans, D. L. (1992). Coping with the treat of AIDS: The role of social support. *American Journal of Psychiatry, 149*, 1514-20.

Namir, S., Wolcott, D., Fawzy, F., & Alumbaugh, M. (1990). Implications of different strategies for coping with AIDS. *Psychological perspectives of AIDS*. Hillsdales N J: Erlbaum associates.

Orley, J., & Kuyken, W. (Eds.) (1994). *Quality of life Assessment: International Perspectives*. Heidelberg: Springer Verlag.

Rabkin, J. G., Remien, R., Kattoff, L., & Williams, J. B. (1993). Residence in adversity among long time survivors of AIDS. *Hospital Community Psychiatry, 44*, 162-7.

Szabo, S. on behalf of the WHOQOL Group (1996). The World Health Organisation Quality of Life (WHOQOL) Assessment Instrument. In B. Spilker (Ed.) *Quality of Life and Pharmacoeconomics in Clinical Trials* (2nd edition). Philadelphia: Lippincott-Raven Publishers.

Tocco, J. (2009). ARVs, Islamic healing and efficacy beliefs in Northern Nigeria. Paper presented at Conference on Prolonging Life, Challenging Religion April 15-17, 2009 Justo Mwale Colege, Lusaka, Zambia.

Watchel, T., Piette, J., Mor, V., Stein, M., Fleishman, J., & Carpenter, C. (1992). Quality of life in persons with human immunodeficiency infection; management by the medical outcomes study instrument. New York: Oxford university press. *Annals International Medicine, 116,* 129-37

WHO QOL-BREF (1996). Introduction, administration, scoring and generic version of the assessment.

WHOQOL user manual. (2012.3). Programme on mental health. Division of mental health and substance abuse. WHO/HIS/HIS Rev.

HIV/AIDS Knowledge and the Implications for Health Promotion Programs among Adolescents

Dr. Shalini Singh[13], Richa Varshney[14], Dr. Uma Joshi[15]

ABSTRACT

Present study on adolescents regarding HIV/AIDS knowledge and the implication for health promotion programs was conducted in Ghaziabad City. HIV/AIDS is most popular disease and increasing day by day. HIV/AIDS knowledge is limited among the general population in India, lack of knowledge among adolescents might be more alarming than lack of knowledge in the general population because one would expect that adolescents, as future leaders of the society and as educated individuals would be the most knowledgeable about HIV/AIDS.

For the presents study, 50 boys and 50 girls were selected randomly and were interviewed by self-constructed questionnaire. Data was analyzed by percentile technique and results indicate that both boys and girls have knowledge about HIV/AIDS but are not much aware about modes of transmission, symptoms, treatment and preventive measure. The data underscore the urgent need for HIV/AIDS related health promotion and prevention efforts targeting adolescents.

Keywords: HIV/AIDS, Health Promotion Program, Adolescents

World is a beautiful place and so is the experience of living in it, it would be tragic if this beautiful experience of living life is shortened by HIV/AIDS, when its prevention is within one's control, though not the cure. "AIDS is the Acquired Immune Deficiency Syndrome, where as HIV is the Human Immune Deficiency Virus. HIV is the virus that causes the disease that is called 'AIDS". AIDS has no cure

---

[13] Lecturer, Dept. Of H.Sc. V.M.L.G. (P.G.) College, Ghaziabad
[14] Research Scholar, V.M.L.G. (P.G.) College, Ghaziabad
[15] Reader, Dept. Of H.Sc. V.M.L.G. (P.G.) College, Ghaziabad

and its effect is the ultimate death of the infected person (WHO, 1985).

In India people in the age group of 15 -29 yrs comprise almost 25 percent of the country's population however, they account for 31 percent of AIDS burden.This clearly indicates that young people are at high risk of contracting HIV infection. There are now roughly 34 million people living with HIV/AIDS worldwide, out of which 2.5 million people are from India, according to officials, HIV/AIDS prevalence rate in Delhi is 0.21 percent of the total population and more than 15 million children have lost one or both parents to AIDS.

Adolescents and HIV/AIDS

Approximately one billion people-nearly one out of every six persons on the planet-are adolescents. According to WHO estimates, half of the world's HIV infection is found in adolescents, and youth between 15 and 24 years of age. Girlsand young women are highly vulnerable to HIV/AIDS, and lack of education makes them so. Girls and women face heavier risks of HIV infection than men because their diminished economics and social status compromises their ability to choose safer and healthier life strategies (Mishra, 2005). Women forcibly exposed to HIV infection, for example rape and are being denied their right to life. Many socio, cultural and economic factors restrict women's right to health and right to access to health care facilities, further increasing their vulnerability to HIV (Singh, 2005). This is the time when they get interested in sexual relationships. Immature reproductive tracts make them more susceptible to HIV/AIDS. Discussing sex has also been a taboo among them. With the influence of media and the breakdown of traditional family structures, and in the absence of organized institutions for imparting sex education, they tend to learn about sexual and reproductive health from unreliable sources resulting in perpetuation of myths regarding safe sex and reproductive health.

OBJECTIVE

To assess the knowledge and implications for health promotion programs regarding HIV/AIDS among adolescents.

METHODOLOGY

Multistage stratified random sampling technique was used for selection of samples. Ghaziabad City has been selected purposively as it is convenient to the researcher. Total sample was 100 (boys-50, girls-50) were selected. A self constructed interview-cum-questionnaire schedule was prepared by researcher and administered on adolescents. Analysis of data was done by percentile technique.

RESULT AND DISCUSSION-

The collected data was tabulated and the results obtained are presented under the following tables:-

Table 1: Distribution of respondents according to source of information regarding HIV/AIDS

Source of Information	Male (n=50)	Female (n=50)	Total (n=100)
Television	40%	50%	45%
Radio	32%	15%	46%
Newspaper	22%	8%	30%
Road side play	14%	10%	15%
NGO	12%	3%	15%
Friend	24%	6%	31%

Table 2: Distribution of respondents according to awareness regarding modes of transmission of HIV/AIDS

Modes of Transmission	No. of aware students (%)		
	Male (n=50)	Female (n=50)	Total (n=100)
Unprotected sexual intercourse	54%	24%	78%
Homosexual intercourse	22%	6%	26%
Infected Blood transfusion	52%	19%	72%
Sharing needles/syringes/blades	56%	19%	76%
HIV infected Mother to baby	39%	15%	54%

Table 3: Distribution of respondents according to myths regarding HIV/AIDS

Myths	No. of students with 'Yes' Responses (%)		
	Male (n=50)	Female (n=50)	Total (n=100)
Mosquito bite can spread HIV/AIDS	15%	6%	21%
HIV/AIDS can spread through kissing	15%	4%	18%
HIV/AIDS can spread through touching an infected person	11%	4%	14%
Sharing same clothes can spread HIV/AIDS	10%	5%	14%
Eating together can spread HIV/AIDS	13%	6%	19%
Living together canspread HIV/AIDS	12%	4%	16%
HIV/AIDS canspread throughcommon/publictoilet	9%	3%	12%

Table 4: Distribution of respondents according to awareness regarding methods of prevention of HIV/AIDS

Methods of Prevention	No. of Aware Students (%)		
	Male (n=50)	Female (n=50)	Total (n=100)
Using condom during each Intercourse	60%	20%	79%
Not having sex with prostitute	35%	8%	42%
Having a single sexual partner	48%	12%	60%
Abstaining from homosexual Intercourse	23%	4%	26%
Screening of blood prior to transfusion	53%	23%	73%
Using sterilized/disposable syringes	53%	17%	69%

Table 5: Attitude of respondents towards people with HIV/AIDS

Responses (Yes)	Male (n=50)	Female (n=50)	Total (n=100)
Awareness regarding the difference between HIV +ve and AIDS	31%	10%	40%
Awareness regarding the symptoms of AIDS	31%	9%	39%
Knowledge about HIV/AIDS being cured	32%	21%	52%
PLWHA should be kept separate, isolated from others	25%	15%	39%
PLWHA should be socially supported, sympathized and cared	34%	14%	48%

CONCLUSION

In the present study all the students had heard about HIV/AIDS. These observations show the strength and effectiveness of media as source of information and very poor effort by health personnel which requires being strongly motivated. The awareness regarding modes of transmission and methods of prevention of HIV/AIDS was found to be significantly higher among boys as compared to girls. Thus adolescent girls lacked awareness regarding HIV/AIDS. 59% females indicating that HIV transmission could be prevented by using condom. 79% students thought that use of condom decrease the risk of getting AIDS. Study revealed that 20.5% of the students believed that mosquito bite could transmit the disease while 18.2% students thought that it could spread by sharing meals. In the current study 59.5% students stated that HIV/AIDS can be prevented by having a single sexual partner. Only 39.6% students in our study knew that HIV and AIDS are not synonymous.

SUGGESTIONS

Adolescents need to be taught about the body functions since ignorance perpetuates myths and mis-belief. School teachers play a key role in bringing about this desirable change and serially acceptable approaches to sex education such as letterbox approach may be used for providing scientific knowledge about sex and related issues. The challenge lies in developing programmes to spread awareness and to induce behavioral changes among them. The School Adolescent Education Programme has been focused to create awareness of HIV/AIDS and to inform adolescents, about the dangerous consequences of unsafe sex and encouraging them to use condoms.

REFERENCES

Chakrovarty A, Nandy S, Roy R, Sengupta B, Chatterjee S, and Chaudhari RN. A study of awareness on HIV/AIDS among higher secondary school students incentral Kolkata. Indian Journal of Community Medicine 2007; 32(3):228-229.

Goyal R C: Community based study on demographic: Health and psychological profile and needs of the people living with HIV/AIDS in rural areas of Ahmad Nagar district in Maharashtra. Indian Journal of Medical Research, 2003, 22(1) 49-53.

Khadilkar HA, Warkari PD, Yadav VB, Soundale SG. Impact of health education on knowledge about HIV/AIDS among students of social sciences. Indian Journal of Community Medicine 2005; 30 (4):150.

Lal P, Nath A, Badhan S, Ingle GK. A study of awareness about HIV/AIDS among senior secondary school children of Delhi. Indian Journal of Community Medicine 2008; 33 (3):190-192.

MHRD (2004) Selected Educational Statistics 2003-04. Ministry of Human Resource Development, Govt. of India.

Singh A and Jain S. Awareness of HIV/AIDS among school adolescents in anaskantha district of Gujarat. Health and Population: Perspectives and Issues 2009; 32 (2):59-65,

UNAIDS. Report on the global AIDS epidemic.UNAID: Geneva; 2007.

HIV: A Psychological Consequence

Miss. Sana Akhter[16]

ABSTRACT

There are number of consequences of HIV/AIDS but in this paper reviews the literature on psychological consequences. HIV is a significantly related to Psychological problems like mental health problem, including substance-use disorders, depression and anxiety, post-traumatic stress disorder (PTSD), suicide and coping, cognitive disorders (including dementia), psychotic disorders, disorders of personality can influence behavior, memory disturbance, concentration problems and slowness of thinking as symptoms that are reported more often by individuals with HIV-related symptoms. People with HIV often suffer from depression and anxiety as they adjust to the impact of the diagnosis of being infected and face the difficulties of living with a chronic life-threatening illness, for instance shortened life expectancy, complicated therapeutic regimens, stigmatization, and loss of social support, family or friends. HIV infection can be associated with high risk of suicide or attempted suicide. The psychological predictors of suicidal ideation in HIV-infected individuals include concurrent substance-use disorders, past history of depression and presence of hopelessness. Treisman et al. claim that most HIV positive psychiatric patients actually suffer from multiple disorders. They classify these disorders into the following four categories, this appear in the American Psychiatric Association's Diagnostic and Statistical Manual of Mental Disorders, Fourth Edition (DSM-IV). (i) Problems that Emerge from Life Circumstances, (ii) Brain Diseases, (iii) Personality and Temperament Disorders and (iv) Disorders of Motivated Behavior. HIV infection has direct effects on the central nervous system, and causes neuropsychiatric complications including HIV encephalopathy, depression, mania, cognitive disorder, and frank dementia, often in combination. Infants and children with HIV infection are more likely to experience

---

[16] Research Scholar, Kolhan University, Chaibasa

deficits in motor and cognitive development compared with HIV negative children.

Keywords: *HIV/AIDS, Psychological Consequences, People Living with HIV/AIDS (PLWHA)*

AIDS the acquired immune deficiency syndrome is a fatal illness caused by a retrovirus virus known as the human immune deficiency virus (HIV) which breaks down the body's immune system, learning the victim vulnerable to a host of life threatening opportunistic infections, neurological disorders or unusual malignancies. Among the special features of HIV infection are that once infected, it is portable that a person will be infected for life. Strictly speaking the term AIDS refer only the last stage of the HIV infection (WHO, 2002).

HIV/AIDS is a global epidemic and it is a significant cause of death and disability. HIV Positive People have facing many psychological consequences. HIV is a chronic stressor that places HIV-infected persons as well as their immediate and extended families at risk for psychological distress and psychiatric disorders. Because patients and their families may have histories of substance use, chronic mental illness, poverty, physical abuse, violence, and isolation, they may have limited coping skills. Chandra et, al.(2015) state that HIV infection and psychiatric disorders have a complex relationship. Being HIV infected could result in psychiatric disorders as a psychological consequence of the infection or because of the effect of the HIV virus on the brain. Disorders may be as varied as depression, post-traumatic stress disorders, AIDS phobias, grief and the whole gamut of cognitive disorders. In addition, several psychiatric conditions may predispose individuals to acquiring HIV infection as a consequence of their influence on behaviour. There is also strong evidence of the relationship of substance use disorders and severe mental illnesses with HIV infection. HIV related

90

psychiatric disorders also offer a challenge to clinicians in issues of differential diagnosis and management. Majority of the work in India has focused on substance use and HIV, and to a lesser extent on the psychiatric effects of HIV infection. Given the magnitude of the problem in the country and the multiple physical and psychological stressors that persons with HIV face in India, more research is needed. Because most patients with HIV and mental illness are seen in primary care settings, primary care practitioners are often the first to assess the risk of mental distress and to observe its signs and symptoms. These psychiatric disorders include:

- Mood disorders
- Substance use
- Personality disorders
- Adjustment disorders
- Cognitive disorders
- Depression
- Suicide risk
- Anxiety disorders

REVIEW OF LITERATURE

HIV/AIDS has no age-appropriateness and not even children are spared. In the Namibian context, an orphan is a child who has lost one or both parents or guardians to HIV/AIDS before reaching the age of 18, and who remains dependent (Sr. Mallmann, Catholic Aids Action, 2002).

HIV infections continue to increase rapidly among women, who made up 22 percent of cases in the U.S. in 1997 and now make up 42% percent of cases worldwide. (www.HIV+standard of women 2005).

There are a number of psychological impacts affecting children of HIV/AIDS parents. A parent who is HIV infected may show less interest in the child due to the dramatic mood swings associated with the pressure of being infected. The child usually does not know what the problem is, that it is not his or her fault, and does not understand why the parent seems moody. The child is likely to react with fear and anxiety and sometimes will blame themselves (Sr. Mallmann, Catholic Aids Action, 2002).

The psychosocial impacts of stress, grief, avoidance and teasing by other children, social isolation and discrimination can lead to behavioral disturbances, fatalism, self-stigmatization, and increased opportunities for abuse (Claudia Tjikuua, 2002).

Researchers have observed symptoms associated with trauma, depression and lack of bonding and attachment in very young children. This may lead to children feeling deprived of their childhood, causing misery and sometimes thoughts of suicide. Access to experiences which address psychosocial needs such as consistency of care appeared to be unmet for many children (C.K. Haihambo, 2004).

Many orphans are usually incorporated into the extended families that act as a safety net. However the shrinking number of caregivers and the considerable strain on families means that children are much more vulnerable to economic and social hardships such as malnutrition, poverty, child labour, homelessness and reduced access to education and healthcare (AIDS brief, 2004).

Low Beer et. al., (2000) found that as many as one half of HIV infected persons significant levels of depression making depression a particularly important factor in determining health and in HIV-infected women's evaluation of their health.

Voss et. al., (2007) fatigue and depression are among the most frequently rated symptoms of people with HIV/AIDS women experienced higher fatigue and depression severity scores than men.

PURPOSE

The purpose of this paper is to extend knowledge about HIV/AIDS and their psychological consequence such as: fear, loss, grief, guilt, anger, anxiety, low self-esteem, depression, suicidal behavior and thinking, and psychological disorder.

MATERIALS AND METHODS

The contents have been taken from relevant books and articles, research paper, forms journals and website. The method used is theoretical, and no practical work has done.

RESULTES AND DISSCATION

"The psychological or internal challenges a person with HIV/AIDS faces vary from individual to individual. Not everyone will experience all of the emotional responses or stages of the emotional responses described. Each HIV/AIDS situation is as unique as the people involved. There are individuals who might face catastrophic changes not only in their personal and job relationships, but in their physical bodies and in their self-images and self-esteem." (Watstein and Chandler, 1998).

Infected persons are normally in fear because they have to adjust to a new lifestyle. It is not easy to accept that one is infected and thus shock and disbelief, leading to denial, is a frequent initial response. According to Watstein and Chandler (1998) there are emotional responses that are symptoms of the psychological effects that people have when infected or affected with HIV/AIDS. Watstein and Chandler continue to explain that another destructive stressor is that of feeling dependent. The dependency occurs when the infected person must rely heavily on family and friends for emotional and financial support, particularly when they have to apply for social services assistance.

NEUROPSYCHIATRIC AND PSYCHOLOGICAL DISORDERS ASSOCIATED WITH HIV/AIDS

The World Health Organization asserts that the mental health consequences of AIDS are "substantial."(World Health Organization) In addition to general emotional responses of "anger, guilt, fear, denial, and despair," Lucia Gallego et al,. (2000) 38 to 73 percent of HIV/AIDS patients will have at least one psychiatric disorder in their lifetimes,(Gallego, Gordillo and Catalan) with up to 20 percent of PLWHA exhibiting psychiatric symptoms as their earliest medical symptoms of AIDS(Robert A. Stern et al., -2000). Mental disorders associated with HIV/AIDS can result from the psychological impact of having a fatal disease, or stem from the effects of psychosocial stressors associated with the illness like stigma and discrimination. They can also result from actual neurological changes in the physical and chemical structures of the central nervous system that occur as a result of the HIV virus, opportunistic infections, or related treatments (Stern, Perkins, and Evans). Treisman et al. claim that most HIV positive psychiatric patients actually suffer from multiple disorders. They classify these disorders into the following four categories, described and elaborated below (Glenn J. Treisman-2001). Most of the disorders discussed in this section appear in the American Psychiatric Association's Diagnostic and Statistical Manual of Mental Disorders, Fourth Edition (DSM-IV).

1. Problems that Emerge from Life Circumstances
2. Brain Diseases
3. Personality and Temperament Disorders
4. Disorders of motivated behavior

1. Problems that Emerge from Life Circumstances

HIV/AIDS infected individuals face a number of the same stressors confronted by other patients with chronic illness, such as long-term discomfort, physical deterioration, physical and financial dependence and eventual death. These factors contribute to higher mental disorder prevalence among chronically ill people (30-50%) than among the general population (15-30%),(Gallego, Gordillo and Catalan) and suicide rates that are 7 to 37 times the rates of demographically comparable groups(Stern, Perkins and Evans). Disorders resulting from life circumstances may take the form of adjustment disorder, which is also known as demoralization. Demoralization has many of the same symptoms as depression, including sadness, feelings of helplessness, and sleep disturbances, but is treated through psychotherapy, not medication(Treisman, Angelino and Hutton).For HIV/AIDS patients, demoralization generally springs from the strain of chronic illness, social stigma, and the process of accepting mortality. Acutestress is also common for PLWHA immediately following an HIV positive diagnosis and as new symptoms develop(José Catalán, Adrian Burgess and IvanaKlimes,). In addition to emotional reactions, acute stress can lead to "somatic symptoms, suicidal ideation" and "substance abuse."(Gallego, Gordillo and Catalan).

HIV/AIDS-related stressors can elicit high levels of anxiety among PLWHA. Anxiety may manifest itself through motor symptoms like shakiness and jumpiness, autonomic responses such as palpitations, excessive sweating, hyperventilation, rapid heartbeat, and diarrhea, or vigilance symptoms including hypervigilance, decreased sleep, irritability and distractibility (Warren and Stern, Anxiety Disorders). Anxiety can also be a symptom of other AIDS-related mental disorders like depression (Warren and Stern).

2. Brain Diseases

Neuropsychiatric disorders in HIV/AIDS patients are often overlooked since psychiatric are frequently misconstrued as psychological in nature (E. Koutsilieri, et al.,). However, actual neurological impairment can occur as a direct effect of HIV/AIDS on the central nervous system

(CNS) or result from opportunistic infections that the body is defenseless against due to immune system damage.147,148(Tiffany A. Chenneville and Howard M. Knoff-2004, F. Daniel Armstrong, John F. Seidel and Thomas P. Swales-1993) Brain diseases typically manifest themselves in syndromal forms and are caused by "structural or functional brain lesions"(Treisman, Angelino and Hutton). Autopsies reveal that three-fourths of all HIV/AIDS patients experience neurological changes, and 30 percent exhibit multiple lesions in the CNS(Stern, Perkins, and Evans).Examples of common, HIV/AIDS-related brain disorders include AIDS Dementia Complex (ADC), tumors, and opportunistic infections such as TB and cryptococcal meningitis.

3. Personality and Temperament Disorders

Treismen et al. cite two personality dimensions that are critical considerations in HIV/AIDS patient treatment. The first, stability-instability, looks at how patients react to and cope emotionally with stimuli (Treisman, Angelino and Hutton). For example, unstable patients are more likely to react to adverse situation with strongly negative emotions that may further compromise their health. In the second dimension, introversion-extroversion, extroverts "tend to seek rewards rather than avoid consequences" and "focus on the present rather than the future" (Treisman, Angelino and Hutton). Introverts, conversely, are more concerned with consequences. Though there are strengths and weaknesses associated with each trait, HIV/AIDS patients who tend toward instability and extroversion exhibit a higher level of risky behavior, have worse adherence to treatment regimens, and have more problems coping with the disease than their more stable, introverted peers (Treisman, Angelino and Hutton).

4. Disorders of motivated behavior

Research shows that 20 to 73 percent of HIV/AIDS infected individuals have substance abuse Disorders(Gallego, Gordillo and Catalan). In fact, transmission through injected drug use currently accounts for 5 percent of worldwide HIV infection(UNAIDS, "World AIDS Campaign 2001 Fact Sheet."). For some, the mechanics of the substance use disorder (i.e.injection) or the impaired judgment and impulsivity associated with drug or alcohol use led to HIV infection. For others, substance abuse is a coping mechanism for dealing with an HIV positive diagnosis. It is critical that substance abuse disorders in the general population and among PLWHA be addressed since users are "prone to have sexual behaviors at risk for HIV transmission" due to "a higher rate of sexual dis-inhibition, impaired judgment, and impulsivity"(Gallego, Gordillo and Catalan).

Social support is an important determinant of health for PHAs (Borgoyne& Renwick, 2004; Richmond, Ross, & Egeland, 2007). Greater levels of social support have been shown to increase the number of visits a patient makes to a doctor's office (Tamers, Beresford, Thompson, Zheng, & Cheadie, 2011), decrease stress, and increase physical (Moak & Agrawal, 2010) and mental health outcomes (Richmond et al., 2007; Bekele et al., 2013). Indeed, the availability of social support in PHAs is an integral part of achieving and maintaining optimal quality of life (Broadhead et al., 1983).

CONCLUSION

There are many Psychological Consequences of HIV/AIDS. Psychological interventions have been shown to increase the quality of life substantially for PLWHA (Catalan, 151-160).They can also play an important role in reducing the transmission of HIV by persons infected with the virus, especially adolescents and young adults. As antiretroviral medications become more widely used and prolong life for these young people, the risks of them handling life's normal frustrations and disappointments inappropriately and deliberately exposing others to the infection may also increase. With this in mind, developing culturally appropriate psychological interventions that target the young is critical. Such interventions could help them to cope better with their infection status, build the skills necessary for self-disclosure, and improve self-esteem. They should also address strategies for staying healthy with HIV, preventing future transmission, avoiding substance abuse, and moving forward with life (Catalan, 151-156).The interventions could be offered by primary care clinicians and others involved in the management of PLWHA (OyeGureje).

REFERENCES

"AIDS Brief",Nabcoa's Quarterly Publication, 2004

Bekele, T., Rourke, S.B., Tuckler, R., Greene, S., Sobota, M., Joornstra, J., Monette, L., Reuda, S., Bacon, J., Watson, J., Hwang, S.W., Dunn, J., Guenter, D. (2013). Direct and indirect effects of perceived social support on health-related quality of life in persons living with HIV/AIDS.AIDS Care, 25(3): 337-346.

Borgoyne, R., Renwick, R. (2004). Social Support and Physical Health.SocSci Med, 58(7): 1353-1266.

Broadhead, W.E., Kaplan, B.H., James, S.A., Wagner, E.H., Schoenbach, V.J., Grimson, R., Heyden, S., Tibblin, G., Gehlbach, S.H. (1983). The Epidemiological Evidence for a Relationship between Social Support and Health.Am J Epidemiol, 117(5): 521-537.C.K. Haihambo, An Assessment of Services Provided to Children Infected and Affected by HIV/AIDS in Windhoek, Namibia, 2004

Calvert Warren and Robert Stern, "Neuropsychiatric Emergencies in the Patient with HIV Infection," Emergency Medicine Reports 16, no. 15 (24 July 1995), epidemiology.

Catalán, José, Adrian Burgess and IvanaKlimes.Psychological Medicine of HIV Infection. Oxford: Oxford University Press, 1995.

Catalan, Jose. "Psychological Interventions." In Mental Health and HIV Infection: Psychological and Psychiatric Aspects. Edited by Jose Catalan, 151-163. London: University College London,1999.

Claudia Tjikuua,"Impacts of HIV/AIDS on Education in Namibia", Presentation speech by Chief Education Officer, 2002

E. Koutsilieri, et al., "Psychiatric Complications in Human Immunodeficiency Virus Infection," Journal of NeuroVirology8, no. 2 (2002): 129.

F. Daniel Armstrong, John F. Seidel and Thomas P. Swales, "Pediatric HIV Infection: A Neuropsychological and Educational Challenge," Journal of Learning Disabilities 26, no.2 (February 1993): 93.

Gallego, Lucia, Victoria Gordillo, and Jose Catalan. "Psychiatric and Psychological Disorders associated to HIV Infection." AIDS Reviews 2, no. 1 (2000): 48-60.

Glenn J. Treisman, Andrew F. Angelino, and Heidi E. Hutton, "Psychiatric Issue in the Management of Patients with HIV Infection," Journal of the American Medical Association 286, no. 22 (21 December 2001): 2857. HIV+: standard of care: women (2005) www.HIV/women.htm

Low-Beer, S., Chan, K., Yip,B. Wood, E., Montaver, J.S., O'Shaughnessy, M.V., & Hogg, R.S. (2000). Depressive symptoms decline among persons on HIV protease inhibitors. Journal of Acquired Immune Deficiency Syndrome, 23, 295-301.

Moak, Z.B., Agrawal, A. (2010). The Association between perceived interpersonal social support and physical and mental health: results from the national epidemiological survey on alcohol and related conditions. J Public Health, 32(2): 191-201.

OyeGureje, Professor and Head of the Department of Psychiatry University Of Ibadan, Nigeria, comments to authors.

PrabhaS.Chandra, Geetha Desai* &Sanjeev Ranjan-2005, HIV & psychiatric disorders, Indian J Med Res 121, April 2005, pp 451-467.

Richmond, C.A., Ross, N.A., Egeland, G.M. (2007). Social Support and Thriving Health: A New Approach to Understanding the Health of Indigenous Canadians. Am J Public Health,7(9): 1827 – 1833.

Robert A. Stern, Diana O. Perkins, and Dwight L. Evans, "Neuropsychiatric Manifestations of HIV-1 Infection and AIDS," in Psychopharmacology. The Fourth Generation of Progress, eds. F. E. Bloom and D. J. Kupfer. New York: Raven Press Ltd, 2000.

S.B.Watstein, K. Chandler, The AIDS Dictionary. Facts on File, Inc.New York, 1998.

Sr. Silke-Andrea Mallman, Building Resiliency Among Children Affected by HIV/AIDS,Windhoek, Catholic AIDS Action Claudia Tjikuua,"Impacts of HIV/AIDS on Education in Namibia", Presentation speech by Chief Education Officer, 2002

Tamers, S.L.; Beresford, S.A., Thompson, B., Zheng, Y., Cheadie, A.D. (2011). Exploring the role of co-worker social support on health care utilization and sickness absence. JOccup Environ Med, 53(7) 751-757.

Tiffany A. Chenneville and Howard M. Knoff, "HIV/AIDS: What Parents Should Know,"

National Mental Health and Education Center, 1998, <http://www.naspcenter.org/adol_HIV.html> (14 August 2004), Neurological Implications.

UNAIDS."World AIDS Campaign 2001 Fact Sheet."<http://www.thebody.com/unaids/ pdfs/fs_wac.pdf> (20 August 2004).

Voss, J. (2007.) symptoms cluster of fatigue and depression in HIV/AIDS Preventive intervention community, 33 (1-2), 19-34. Abstract

WHO. (2002). AIDS watch, news from WHO SEAR on STD. AIDS and Tuberculosis, 5(1).

World Health Organization. Atlas: Mental Health Resources in the World. Geneva: WHO, 2001

Emotional Maturity and HIV/AIDS Care Awareness of Working and Non-Working Woman

Irfan Khan GulamNabi Makrani[17]

ABSTRACT

The Present research has done to know the effect and care awareness of Working and Non-Working Women on Emotional Maturity and HIV AIDS Care. For this research are Total number of sample was 60 in which 30 working women from the age group of 20 to 40 years. And 30 non-working women were taken the same age group. For the data collection Emotional maturity scale developed by Roma Pal (1988) and AIDS care awareness inventory was used for data analysis and concluded result t test was used. For this dimension implies that in positive sense there was significant difference between working and non-working women. The result indicate the working women significantly differ on Emotional maturity score as compared to non-working women and AIDS Care awareness Score as compare to non-working woman. Working women have shown better Emotional Maturity and AIDS care awareness compared to non-working women.

Keywords: HIV/AIDS, Emotional Maturity

Emotion is the complex psycho physiological experience of an individual's state of mind as interaction with biochemical (internal) and environmental (external) influences. In humans, emotion fundamentally involves "physiological arousal, expressive behaviors and conscious experience." Emotion is associated with mood, temperament, personality, disposition, and motivation. Motivations direct and energize behavior, while emotions provide the affective component to motivation, positive or negative. A

---

[17] Professor in Psychology, Gacc Jadar

related distinction is between the emotion and the results of the emotion, principally behaviors and emotional expressions. People often behave in certain ways as a direct result of their emotional state, such as crying, fighting or fleeing. If one can have the emotion without a corresponding behavior, then we may consider the behavior not to be essential to the emotion.

HIV/AIDS related is invoked as a persistent and pernicious problem in any discussion about effective responses to the epidemic. In addition to devastating the familial, social, and economic lives of individuals, H/A stigma is cited as a major barrier to accessing prevention, care, and treatment services. Despite widespread recognition of the differential treatment of persons living with HIV/AIDS by society and its institutions, over the first 25 years of the epidemic, community, national, and global actors have only had limited success in alleviating the deleterious effects of H/A stigma. In describing a sustained response to the HIV/AIDS epidemic, Peter Piot, Executive Director of UNAIDS, identifies tackling stigma and discrimination as one of five key imperatives for success. At the same time, Piot notes that stigma reduction efforts are relegated to the bottom of AIDS program priorities, often without funding to support such activities. Much of the rhetoric and literature has cited the complexity of H/A stigma and its diversity in different cultural settings as the primary reasons for the limited response to this pervasive phenomenon The complexity of the phenomenon has led to difficulties and disagreement about how to define H/A stigma and sometimes, to an erroneous conflation of stigma with its related concept of discrimination. The manifestation of H/A stigma not only varies by cultural/national setting, but also by whether one is considering intrapersonal versus societal levels of stigma. The variability in manifestations of stigma by setting and level has led to difficulty in measuring the extent of stigma, assessing the impact of stigma on the effectiveness of HIV prevention/treatment programs, and devising interventions to reduce stigma. These four challenges –

defining, measuring, assessing impact of, and reducing stigma – among others have hampered local and global efforts to address H/A stigma.In this paper, we systematically review the scientific literature on H/A stigma to document the current state of research, with an emphasis on identifying gaps in as well as summarizing existing knowledge on the four aforementioned challenges to effective intervention–defining, measuring, assessing impact of, and reducing stigma. In assessing impact, we critically examine the literature to elucidate the relationship of H/A stigma to the effectiveness of HIV prevention and treatment programs. Finally, based on the available literature, we offer recommendations for each of the four challenges that we believe represent critical next steps in ameliorating the devastating effects of H/A stigma

REVIEW OF RELATED LITERATURE

According to Gole man (1995), we have two minds, one that thinks and one that feels, these two fundamentally different ways of knowing, interact to construct our mental life. The rational mind is the mode of comprehension we are typically conscious of more prominent in awareness, thoughtful, able to ponder and reflect. The emotional mind is impulsive and powerful and sometimes illogical. These two minds operate in harmony with each other, most of times feelings are essential to thought, and most of the times thoughts to feeling. But when passions surge the balance tips: it is not just I.Q., but emotional intelligence that matters. Goleman rightly points out that, "It is not that we want to do away with emotions and put reason in its place, but instead find an intelligent balance of two .According to Walter DSmitson (1974) emotional maturity is a process in which thepersonality is continuously striving for greater sense of emotional health, both intra physicallyand intra-personally.Kaplan and Baron elaborate the characteristics of an emotionally mature person say that he has the capacity to withstand delay in satisfaction of needs. He has the ability to tolerate a reasonable amount of frustration. He has belief in long-term planning and is capable of delaying or revising his expectations in terms of demands of situations. An emotionally mature child has the capacity to make effective adjustment with himself, members of his family and his peers in the school, society and culture. But maturity means not merely the capacity for such attitude and functioning but also the ability to enjoy them fully there are many various factors are put its effect on Emotional Maturity one of them is women. Present research is done to know that effect of working and non-working women on Emotional Maturity.

The prevalence of AIDS in India in 2013 was 0.27, which is down from 0.41 in 2002.While the National AIDS Control Organisation estimated that 2.39 million people live with HIV/AIDS in India in 2008–09,a more recent investigation by the Million Death Study Collaborators in the British Medical Journal (2010) estimates the population to be between 1.4–1.6 million people.

Problems of study
The problem of the present study is as under –
Emotional Maturity and HIV AIDS Care Awareness of Working and Non-Working Woman
Objectives of the study
The main objectives of present study are as under:
1. To study of the Emotional Maturity and AIDS care awareness among working and non - working women.
2. To study and compare the various dimension of Emotional Maturity and AIDS care awareness of working and non - working women.

Hypothesis
The main hypotheses of present study are as under:
1. There is no significant difference between working and non - working women in
2. Various dimension of Emotional Maturity.
3. There is no significant difference between working and non - working women in Emotional Stability
4. There is no significant difference between working and non - working women in Various dimension of AIDS care awareness.

5. There is no significant difference between working and non-working women in AIDS care awareness

6. There is no significant difference between working and non-working women in Emotional Regression.

7. There is no significant difference between working and non - working women in Faulty Social adjustment.

8. There is no significant difference between working and non working women in Lack of Independency.

9. There is no significant difference between working and non-working women in Flexibility.

10. There is no significant difference between working non-working woman in AIDS care awareness

Variables
The variables of present study are having given in following.

Independent variable:
Working and non-working women.

Dependent variable:
Various dimension of Emotional Maturity are measured by Roma Pal (1988)
AIDS Awareness Inventory Punita Govil. PG English

Sample:
The main aim of the present research is "A comparative study of Emotional Maturity and AIDS care awareness of working and non - working women". For this total no of sample were 60 in which 30 working women from the age group of 18 to 40 years. And 30 non -working women were taken from the same age group.

Tool:
Emotional maturity scale developed by Roma Pal (1988) was used to measure emotional maturity the scale contains 40 items with totally agree, neutral, generally, disagree and totally disagree.

Response alternative the responses were marked 5,4,3,2 and 1 respectively and from the responses we had to select only one response in every sentence. 5 for tick mark totally agree, 4 for tick mark agree, 3 for tick mark neutral, 2 for tick mark disagree and 1 for tick mark totally disagree. The maximum possible score is 200 and minimum is 40.Scoring pattern shows that more score indicates less emotional maturity. The fewer score in the scale indicates good (more) emotional maturity. The reliability score of emotional maturity scale comes to 0.84, derived by the split half method, obtained from the sample of 200 students. The researcher of the present research has found out the reliability score as 0.81, by using split-half technique on the sample of 50 students

AIDS Awareness Inventory Punita Govil. PG English(This scale consists 60 items divided into five area–(i) Nature & Symptoms of Disease, (ii)Causes of disease, (iii) Prevention of Disease, (iv) Myths regarding the Disease, (v) Awareness about Disease. Age group 18+)

PROCEDURE

After establishing report Emotional Maturity inventory and AIDS Care awareness inventory were administered individuals to every subject. All the instruction were strictly following which are been given the manual of inventory. The responses of inventory have scored as per scoring keys .This has given in the manual of inventory. The data was categories and arranged in respective table according to the stoical technique appraised.

Statically Analysis

The main aim of the present research is to study and compare to Emotional maturity and AIDS Care awareness between working and non -working women. Scoring was done as per scoring key of the inventory to examine significantly difference between working and non working women. For data analysis „t‟ test was used.

RESULTS

Table: 1 N=60 Show in Mean, SD, and „t" ratio of various group of age on score of various dimensions of mental health Dimension of Emotional Maturity and AIDS Care awareness Group N Mean SD 't' Significant
Level Emotional instability

Variables	Group	N	Mean	SD	't'	Significant
Emotional maturity Emotional instability Emotional Regression	Working Non-working woman	30 30	33.68 30.23	3.3 3.3	3.87	0.01
AIDS care awareness	Working Non-working woman	30 30	27.61	10.61	3.96	

DISCUSSION

In result table an attempt is to find out the different between working and non- working women in various dimension of Emotional Maturity and AIDS care awareness score with „t" test t value of working and non-working women of Emotional instability score is 3.87, which is significant act 0.01 level. It means working women are significant differ on AIDS care awareness Positive score as compare to non - working women. Working women have shown better Emotional instability by getting high mean score M =33.87 then non-working women mean M=30.23 t" value of working and non-working women of AIDS care awareness is 1.46 which is not significant. Working women have shown better by AIDS care awareness getting high mean score M=28.10 then non - working women M=26.67„t" value of working and non -working women of Faulty social adjustment is 2.40 which is significant at

0.05 level. It means working women are significant differ on Faulty emotional maturity score as compare to non -working women. Working women have shown better Faulty by AIDS care awareness getting high mean score M=37.57 then non - working women M=34.23„t" value of working and non -working women of Lack of Independency is 3.01 which is significant at 0.01 level. It means working women are significant differ on Lack of Independency score as compare to non-working women.. Working women have shown better overall Emotional maturity by getting high mean score M=18.70 then non -working women M=17.29.

REFERENCES

Alonzo AA, Reynolds NR. Stigma, HIV, and AIDS: An exploration and elaboration of a stigma trajectory. SocSci Med. 1995;41:303–315.

Arunjoseph(2010). Meaning and definition of emotional maturity. Data retrieved on 11 agu 2011 from http//:arunarun joseph. Blogspot.com 2010 /03/study-of-emotional –maturity and-html.

Arya, A. (1997). Emotional Maturity and values of superior children in family. Fourth survey of research in Education Vol.11, New Delhi: NCERT.

Bond V, Chase E, Angleton P. Stigma, HIV/AIDS prevention, and mother to child transmission in Zambia. Evaluation and Program Planning.2002;25:242–356.

Chesney M, Smith A. Critical delays in testing and care: the potential role of stigma. American Behavioural Scientist.1999;42: 1162–1174.

Coleman,(1994).Definition of emotional maturity. data retrieved on 12 oct 2009,from
ssmrae.com/admin/.../37802308c3531dffab3bddd71e963e04.pdf

Crocker J, Major B, Steel C. Social Stigma. In: Gilbert DT, Fiske ST, editors. The handbook of social psychology.Vol. 2. Boston: McGraw-Hill; 1998. pp. 504–553.

Goffman E. Asylums: Essays on the Social Situation of Mental Patients and Other Inmates. Garden City, NY: Anchor Books; 1961.

Goffman E. Stigma: Notes on the Management of Spoiled Identity. Garden City, NY: Anchor Books; 1963.

Kalichman SC, Simbayi L. HIV testing attitudes, AIDS stigma, and voluntary counseling and testing in a Black township in Cape Town, South Africa. Sexually Transmitted Infections.2003;79:442–447

Link BG, Phelan JC. Conceptualizing stigma.Annu Rev Sociol.2001;27:363–85.

Ogden J, Nyblade L. Common at its core: HIV-related stigma across contexts.International Center for Research on Women (ICRW); 2005.

Parker R, Aggelton P. HIV and AIDS-related stigma and discrimination: a conceptual framework and implications for action. SocialScience& Medicine.2003;57:13–24.

Piot P. AIDS: from crisis management to sustained strategic response. Lancet.2006;368:526–530

Somma D, Bond V. International research workshop on health-related stigma and discrimination. Psychology, Health & Medicine.2006;11:271–276.

Stress aspects in HIV/AIDS Disease

Dr Balaji Deekshitulu P V[18]

ABSTRACT

If this study was to determine the correlation of perceived stress with selected physiological and psychological factors in an HIV-infected, correlations between perceived stress and state and trait anxiety, depression, HIV-related symptoms.

Keywords: *HIV/AIDS, Psychological Factors, Stress, Health Tips*

Human immunodeficiency virus, or HIV, is the virus that causes acquired immune deficiency syndrome (AIDS). The virus weakens a person's ability to fight infections and cancer. People with HIV are said to have AIDS when they develop certain infections or cancers or when their CD4 count is less than 200.

HIV disease is a major source of emotional and physiological stress for those who are infected (Faulstich, 1987). Chronic exposure to stressful events reduces immunity, contributes to increased symptomatology and hastens disease progression to AIDS (van Eck et al., 1996). Further, it appears that the physiological and immunological responses to potentially stressful events are due primarily to the individual's assessment of the event, the perceived stress.

Human immunodeficiency virus (HIV) infection and acquired immune deficiency syndrome (AIDS) is a global epidemic that has been reported from all countries. Worldwide, the rate of infected adults is approximately thirty-seven million, 50% of which are women. It is estimated that two million and five hundred thousand

---

[18] Psychologist & Alternative Medicine (Homeopathy) Practitioner, Sri Balaji Clinic, Tirupati, A.P, India.

children under the age of 15 are living with HIV or AIDS. Transmission cases are injection drugs users (IDUs), and the rest of them are affected by sexual intercourse, blood products, and mother-to-child transmission.

Negative thinking and stigma in society against AIDS lead to many social issues, like physical and mental health problems in affected patients, leading to many difficulties in their useful activities and interests. Infected individuals are so vulnerable to many changes in their whole lives including reduction in self-confidence and self-esteem, decrease in daily functions and social activities, increase in sense of vulnerability, disorganized thinking, and also physical symptoms. Moreover, frequent visits to the doctor, the high cost of drugs, and also the side effects of drugs lead to the reduction of quality of life.

Stress is the physiological response to a stressor, when the body reacts to a challenge. Stress typically describes a negative condition or a positive condition that can have an impact on the person's mental and physical well-being. Long-term or chronic stress weakens the immune system and leads to disease susceptibility and makes the body prone to depression. The most common psychiatric disorder in AIDS patients is depression. Depression is a state of low mood and aversion to activity that can affect a person's thoughts, behavior, feeling, and sense of well-being. Depressed people can feel sad, anxious, empty, hopeless, worried, helpless, and worthless.

Cause

- The HIV infection is caused by the human immunodeficiency virus (HIV).
- After HIV is in the body, it starts to destroy CD4+ cells, which are whiteblood cells that help the body fight infection and disease.

- HIV is spread when blood, semen, or vaginal fluids from an infected person enter another person's body, usually through sexual contact, from sharing needles when injecting drugs, or from mother to baby during birth.

-

Symptoms and Complications of HIV/AIDS :Symptoms of HIV infection appear 2 to 12 weeks after exposure. At this point the virus begins rapidly taking over immune cells in the blood. The symptoms of this phase are flu-like and include:
- diarrhoea
- fatigue or weakness
- fever
- headache
- joint pain
- night sweats
- rash
- swollen glands
- weight loss
- yeast infections (of the mouth or vagina) that last a long time or occur frequently

Table : Psychosocial Factors That Can Have a Negative Effect on Immune Function

PSYCHOLOGICAL ISSUES	BEHAVIORAL ISSUES	MEDICAL ISSUES
Preoccupation with death and dying	Restricted breathing patterns (shallow breathing, unconscious breath-holding)	Repeated exposure to HIV and other infections
Chronic impatience		
Sustained survival stress		
Protracted, unmanaged grieving		Limited capacity for self-care when sick
Clinical depression	Inadequate fluid intake (partial dehydration)	
Lack of purpose and		

goals Lack of self-assertiveness Lack of emotional support (or inability to accept support) Poor coping ability	Poor appetite, eating habits, and/or nutrition Insufficient or disrupted sleep Substance abuse, exposure to toxins Inadequate or inappropriate exercise	Limited involvement in/understanding of HIV-related health issues Passive, uninformed relationship with primary care providers

Stress in HIV Patents

If you are HIV infected, you and your loved ones constantly have to deal with stress. Stress is unique and personal to each of us. When stress does occur, it is important to recognize the fact and deal with it. Some ways to handle stress are discussed below. As you gain more understanding about how stress affects you, you will come up with your own ideas for coping with stress.

Try physical activity. When you are nervous, angry, or upset, try exercise or some other kind of physical activity. Walking, yoga, and gardening are just some of the activities you might try to release your tension.

Take care of yourself. Be sure you get enough rest and eat well. If you are irritable from lack of sleep or if you are not eating right, you will have less energy to deal with stressful situations. If stress keeps you from sleeping, you should ask your doctor for help. Talk about it. It helps to talk to someone about your concerns and worries. You can talk to a friend, family member, counselor, or health care provider. Let it out. A good cry can bring relief to your anxiety, and it might even prevent a headache or other physical problem. Taking some deep breaths also releases tension.

AIDS dementia

HIV/AIDS and some medications for treating HIV may affect your brain. When HIV itself infects the brain, it can cause a condition known as AIDS Dementia Complex (ADC). Symptoms can include the following: 1.Forgetfulness, 2. Confusion, 3.Difficulty paying attention, 4. Slurred speech, 5. Sudden shifts in mood or behaviour, 6. Muscle weakness,7.Clumsiness

If you think you may have ADC:

Don't be afraid to tell your doctor that you think something is wrong. These symptoms can be subtle in the beginning, and telling your care providers about your concerns can help them to diagnose and treat you early.

Keep a notepad with you and write down details about your symptoms whenever they occur. This information can help your doctor to help you.

Build as much support as possible, including friends, family, and health care providers. Although it's possible to treat ADC successfully, it may take a while for some symptoms to go away.

Coping tips

It is completely normal to have an emotional reaction upon learning that you are infected with HIV, such as anxiety, anger, or depression. These feelings do not last forever. As noted above, there are many things that you can do to help take care of your emotional needs. Here are just a few ideas:

1. Talk about your feelings with your doctor, friends, family members, or other supportive people.
2. Try to find activities that relieve your stress, such as exercise or hobbies.

3. Try to get enough sleep each night to help you feel rested.
4. Learn relaxation methods such as meditation, yoga, or deep breathing.
5. Limit the amount of caffeine, nicotine, alcohol, and recreational drugs you use.
6. Eat small, healthy meals throughout the day.
7. Join a support group.

There are many kinds of support groups that provide a place where you can talk about your feelings, help others, and get the latest information about HIV/AIDS. Check with your health care provider for a listing of local support groups.

More specific ways to care for your emotional well-being include various forms of therapy and medication. Used alone or in combination, these may be helpful in dealing with the feelings you are experiencing. Therapy can help you better express your feelings and find ways to cope with your emotions. Medicines that may be able to help with anxiety and depression are also available.

The most important thing to remember is that you are not alone; there are support systems in place to help you, including doctors, psychiatrists, family members, friends, support groups, and other services.

Balbin EG et al, (1999) suggested that the psychoneuroimmunological pathways by which immune and neuroendocrine mechanisms might link psychosocial factors with health and long survival.

Leserman J et al,.(1999)study that the more stress and less social support may accelerate the course of HIV disease progression. Additional study will be necessary to elucidate the mechanisms that underlie these relationships and to determine whether interventions that address stress and social support can alter the course of HIV infection.

Murphy DA et al,.(2000)suggested that the both satisfaction with support and adaptive coping were associated directly with depression in HIV-infected adolescents.

L. Grassi et al,.(2007)significant that the psychological stress was significantly correlated with poor coping mechanisms, maladaptive response to illness, external locus of control and weak social support, but not with medical variables. The implications of these findings are discussed.

KH Basavaraj et al ,.(2010)study that the impact of HIV infection on the dimensions of QOL, including physical and emotional well-being, social support systems, and life roles, has emerged as a key issue for persons infected with HIV.

McIntosh RC, and RosselliM(2012)significant that functional impairment, though to a lesser degree. Coping by avoidance and social isolation predicted more severe mental health outcomes. Spirituality and positive reappraisal predicted greater psychological adaptation than did social support seeking. Despite advancements in anti-retroviral treatment for women, HIV/AIDS symptoms and acute and/or chronic psychosocial stress pose the same threat to behavioral and mental health. In the face of these stressors, positive reframing appears to promote psychological adaptation in a way which may lead to positive health outcomes in women living with HIV/AIDS.

Machtinger E et al.,(2012) The findings demonstrate highly disproportionate rates of trauma exposure and recent PTSD in HIV-positive women compared to the general population of women.

Ilse Elisabeth Plattner (2013)indicate that the threat of HIV creates a cognitive and emotional dilemma, which makes young people prone to engaging in denial to maintain trust in their relationships.

Knowledge about HIV-related dating stress and coping mechanisms can benefit psychological counselling and sexual health education for young people.

T. Jayanthi and Dr. V. Srikanth Reddy (2014) Results revealed that Gender is significantly influencing the stress faced by HIV/AIDS patients due to emotional problems, occupational problems and financial problems. Whereas the influence of Gender on stress faced by HIV/AIDS patients due to family problems, health problems and social problems is not significant.

Zahra M Behboodi et al,.(2015)study that the HIV infection is related with psychiatric disorders. According to the results, women are more vulnerable to depression and anxiety and they need more care. Management of these psychiatric disorders is very important and requires innovative comprehensive approaches.

CONCLUSIONS

Associations between psychological stress and disease have been established, particularly for depression, CVD, and HIV/AIDS. Other areas in which evidence for the role of stress is beginning to emerge include upper respiratory tract infections, asthma, herpes viral infections, autoimmune diseases, and wound healing.16Evidence derived from prospective observational studies provides support for stress as an important factor in certain diseases but cannot establish a causal relationship. However, the review of these studies are consistent with those of natural experiments regarding the effects of real-life stressor exposure on disease risk; with those of laboratory experiments showing that stress modifies disease-relevant biological processes in humans; and with those of animal studies investigating stress as a causative factor in disease onset and progression. This consistency of research findings strongly supports the hypothesis of a causal link. The development of interventions that can reduce the behavioral and biological sequelae of psychological stress and the demonstrated efficacy of such interventions in randomized clinical trials would provide critical data on the clinical importance of this work.

REFERENCES

Balbin EG, Ironson GH, Solomon GF. Ironson GH, Solomon GF.(1999) Stress and coping: the psychoneuroimmunology of HIV/AIDS, Baillieres Best Pract Res Clin Endocrinol Metab.;13(4):615-33.

Basavaraj, MA Navya, R Rashmi(2010) Quality of life in HIV/AIDS, the indian journal; of Sexually Transmitted Disesses and aids Volume : 31 | Issue : 2 | Page : 75-

Faulstich, M. (1987).Psychiatric aspects of AIDS.American Journal of Psychiatry, 144, 551556.

Grassia, G. Caloroa, M. Zamorania & E. Ramelli (2007) Psychological morbidity and psychosocial variables associated with life-threatening illness: A comparative study of patients with HIV infection or cancer, Psychology, Health & Medicine, Volume 2, Issue 1, 29-39.

Jeffrey M. Leiphart, Ph.D. Director of HIV Prevention Services UCSF AIDS Health Project San Francisco, CA. Reprinted from HIV Newsline 4/98.

Ilse Elisabeth Plattner (2013)HIV-related stress in dating relationships and its significance for developmental psychology of adolescence and emerging adulthood, IJP &C, Vol.5(1), pp. 13-22 ,

Leserman J, Jackson ED, Petitto JM, Golden RN, Silva SG, Perkins DO, Cai J, Folds JD, Evans DL.(1999) Progression to AIDS: the effects of stress, depressive symptoms, and social support, Psychosom Med. 1999 May-Jun;61(3):397-406.

McIntosh RC, and RosselliM(2012) Stress and coping in women living with HIV,AIDS Behav. 2012 Nov;16(8):2144-59. doi: 10.1007/s10461-012-0166-5.

Machtinger EL1, Wilson TC, Haberer JE, Weiss DS.(2012) Psychological trauma and PTSD in HIV-positive women, AIDS Behav. 2012 Nov;16(8):2091-100. doi: 10.1007/s10461-011-0127-4.

Murphy DA, Moscicki AB, Vermund SH, Muenz LR.(2000) Psychological distress among HIV(+) adolescents in the REACH study: effects of life stress, social support, and coping. The Adolescent Medicine HIV/AIDS Research Network,J Adolesc Health.;27(6):391-8.

Zahra M Behboodi1, Mina Saadat2, Ebrahim Saadat(2015) Comparison of depression, anxiety, stress, and related factors among women and men with human immunodeficiency virus infection, Journal of Human Reproductive Sciences, Vol. 8, No. 1, January-March, 2015, pp. 48-51

van Eck, M., Berkhof, H., Nicolson, N., & Sulon, J. (1996). The effects of perceived stress, traits, mood states and stressful daily events on salivary cortisol. Psychosomatic Medicine, 58, 447 458.

A Study of Awareness of HIV/AIDS among Adolescents:
(Girls and Boys of Urban and Rural Area)

Dr. Krishna J. Vaghela[19]

ABSTRACT

The purpose of the present study was to examine the awareness level regarding the HIV/AIDS among adolescent youths (girls & boys) of urban and rural area. The sample of two hundred adolescents out of which hundred were girls and hundred were boys both urban and rural area. To measure the HIV/AIDS awareness level of adolescents the HIV/AIDS awareness questionnaire was used. After careful administration of the HIV/AIDS awareness scale, collected information was classified in the light of objectives. On the basis of which certain findings were drawn. There is no significant difference among adolescent girls of urban and rural area towards HIV/AIDS awareness. As regarding the urban and rural area's adolescent boys also found no significant difference regarding to their level of HIV/AIDS awareness.

Keywords: HIV/AIDS, adolescents, girls, boys, area – urban, rural, awareness level.

Acquired Immune Deficiency Syndrome AIDS was unknown in 1980, it has grown explosively in the last twenty years. HIV is now most critical incurable infection in the world. AIDS was first clinically observed in 1981 in the united state. The initial cases were a cluster of injecting drug users and homosexual men with no known cause of impaired immunity who showed symptoms of

---

[19] Asso. Prof. & Head, Deptt. of Psychology, Yogiji Maharaj Mahavidyalaya, Dhari

PNEUMOCYSTIS CARINIL PNEUMONIA PCP a rare opportunistic infection that was known to occur in people with much compromised immune systems. Both HIV – 1 and HIV – 2 are believed to have originated in non-human primates in west central Africa and were transferred to humans in the early 20th century.

The burden of HIV disease has been greatest in the poorest countries, were more than 90% of all HIV infections in children occur. In fact HIV – AIDS is the leading cause of death in Africa, which is home two thirds of people living with, AIDS or HIV and despite intense national and international efforts to control the HIV pandemic more than 16,000 HIV infections occur each day. The spread of HIV promotes poverty and has unleashed immense suffering on different countries and communities worldwide (UNGAS 2001).

HIV human immune deficiency virus is a lent virus (that is a member of the retrovirus family) that causes Acquired Immune Deficiency Syndrome (AIDS) – Doueck, Roededrer, Koup 2009. This is a condition in hernias where the immune system begins to fail leading to life threatening opportunistic infections. AIDS is an incurable fatal disease caused by the human immune deficiency virus (HIV) Wortrman & Loftus 1992. HIV/ AIDS is one of the emerging infections diseases all over the world. The HIV / AIDS is now almost thirty years old and these years millions of people have been infected by HIV.

HIV is now the second most prolific cause of death among young people worldwide. AIDS is spread through contact with the blood, body fluid or semen of an infected person, typically via a blood transfusion or by sharing a needle (in drug use), mother to child transmission (inuteroduring pregnancy, intraparty at childbirth or via breast feeding) or by having sexual contact (whether heterosexual or homosexual) without condom. The receiver partner may be more at risk than the inserting partner. An estimated 3.2 million children were living with HIV at the and of 2013, majority of them acquire HIV from their HIV infected mothers during pregnancy birth or breastfeeding. An estimated 35.3 million people across the world are infected with HIV. The contribution of India to the global burden of HIV/AIDS India is estimated to have the largest burden, with about 3.7 million infection UNAID 2000.

Adolescents and young adults of 15 to 24 years old are the hardest hit by HIV infection worldwide and signification proportion of them live in India. Undoubtedly, the number of HIV positive or AIDS patients is increasing, each of day in the world. In 2013 almost 60% of all new HIV infection among young people aged 15 to 24 occurred among adolescent girls and young women. The young adolescents come in the high risk group because of their propensity to indulge themselves in risky sexual activity and drug abuse. A survey of 1000 adolescents by Diclementc Zorn & Temoshok (1986) found a good deal of confusion about who gets AIDS, how it spreads and how to avoid its infection, even those who know how to protect themselves may not do so, for several reasons.

New studies reveal extremely high level of infections among young girls, which are higher than those for boys. This is mainly because of the face that at young age boys has sex with girls of similar age while girls have relationship with older men who are more likely to be infected (Gregson et. al. 2002). Gupta (2002) asserts that out of every 23 infected people 13 infected are women and this gender gap is especially pronounced among those who are under than 25 years. Fanthum & Chala (1996) found low levels of HIV/AIDS awareness among college students in Ethiopia reporting that a large proportion of their participants do not have accurate knowledge of the causes and prevention of HIV/ AIDS transmission. Ganguli, Pege, Gupta, Charan (2002) in a study on AIDS awareness among undergraduate students Maharashtra and found confusion about mode of transmission and prevention of the disesse exist. Overall knowledge of science students were better compare to commerce and arts students. Ailicky et. al. (2013) in his study on HIV knowledge in high school students in Turkey, revealed a significant gender difference in AIDS knowledge with females being more knowledgeable than males particularly in the areas concerning HIV/AIDS treatment and prevention. Mahajan and Sharma (2005) in a study on awareness level of adolescent girls regarding the HIV/AIDS and found urban adolescent girls have comparatively better knowledge regarding these issues than rural adolescent girls.

Globally, young people have been identified to be at special risk of HIV infection due to their unprotected sexual intercourse and multiple sexual partners. In India Mc Manus and Dhar (2008) in their study of knowledge, perception and attitude of urban adolescent school girls towards HIV in south Delhi, found that them was good awareness about the modes of HIV transmission and prevention among adolescent girls. Bhan et. al. (2004) in a study on awareness regarding sex knowledge on adolescent girls found the awareness regarding HIV/AIDS among adolescent girls is very low. HIV/AIDS infection is rapidly spreading in India unfortunately even in 21st century, awareness of people about the disease is still low. Adolescents need accurate age appropriate information about HIV infection and AIDS, including how to talk with their parents and other trusted adults about HIV and AIDS how to reduce or dominate risk factor how to talk with a potential partner about risk factors, where to get tested for HIV, how to use a condom correctly. There is a strong need to rise the levels of HIV awareness among the young population especially among adolescents. Therefore the current study assessed the awareness level of adolescent girls and boys about HIV/AIDS.

OBJECTIVES:

Briefly the present study was aimed at achieving the following the objectives.

To find out the HIV/AIDS awareness level among adolescent girls of urban and rural area.

To find out the HIV/AIDS awareness level among adolescent boys of urban and rural area.

METHOD:

The present investigation was carried out to study the HIV/AIDS awareness among adolescents (girls & boys) of urban and rural area. The present study was conducted in rural and urban area of Junagadh district in Gujarat. The sample was comprised of 200 adolescent girls and boys in the age group 12 to 17 years. A sample of 100 adolescent girls (50 from rural area and 50 from urban area) and 100 adolescents boys (50 from rural area and 50 from urban area) were selected purposively. And finally 200 adolescents were taken for the assessment of awareness regarding HIV/AIDS through self administered questionnaire. HIV/AIDS awareness questionnaire focused on – Transmission of HIV/AIDS, -Misconception regarding the transmission of HIV/AIDS, - Biological symptoms, - Protection from HIV/AIDS, - Treatment for HIV/AIDS. Necessary instructions were given to participants before administrating the tool. Although the statements were not so difficult to understand, yet necessary assistance was provided to participants where need was felt. All the respondents' adolescents were assured of confidentiality.

Analysis of Data:

To analyze the data, collected information was classified in the light of objectives for the present study the classified data was coded, tabulated and was analyzed by using appropriate statistical technique (t –test).

FINDINGS

The present research paper focuses on the awareness of HIV/AIDS among adolescent girls and boys of urban and rural area. After collecting the data, it is necessary to provide statistical treatment to it so that meaningful information may be drawn out of that. A number of descriptive measures were used to reduce the quantitative data into meaningful and interpretative findings.

The table – 1 reveals that the awareness to modes of transmission of HIV/AIDS in adolescent girls of urban area (38%) and adolescent girls of rural area (24%). Most of the adolescent girls of urban area knew about the misconceptions regarding the mode of HIV/AIDS (43%) and protection from HIV/AIDS (36%). As regarding the awareness of biological symptoms related to HIV/AIDS in adolescent girls of urban area (28%) and rural area (21%). As well as awareness of treatment of HIV/AIDS in adolescent girls of urban area (25%) in rural area adolescent girls (13%) respectively. Table – 1 also reveals that there is no significant difference in the awareness level regarding the HIV/AIDS of adolescent girls of urban area and adolescent girls of rural area were found. It was also observed The lowest level of awareness regarding the treatment of HIV/AIDS in adolescent girls of rural area were noted in the present study. It was also observed that adolescent girls of urban area have the misconception regarding the HIV/AIDS transmission is high in comparison to their rural area's adolescent girls.

Table – 1 Distribution of adolescent girls according to their awareness regarding HIV/AIDS

Respondents (Girls)	Awareness of HIV/AIDS % average score					Total average score	mean score	S.D.	t
	Transmission	Misconception	Biological symptoms	Protection	Treatment				
Urban adolescents	38%	43%	28%	36%	25%	34.00	1.6	1.8	1.01
Rural adolescents	24%	39%	21%	20%	13%	23.4	1.23	1.71	

The table – 2 reveals that the awareness to modes of transmission of HIV/AIDS in adolescent boys of urban area (33%) and adolescent boys of rural area (29%). Most of the adolescent boys of urban area knew about the misconceptions regarding the mode of HIV/AIDS (58%) and awareness of protection from HIV/AIDS (42%). Misconceptions regarding the transmission of HIV/AIDS were noted in the adolescent boys of rural area (61%) and awareness of protection from HIV/AIDS (30%). The misconception regarding HIV/AIDS transmission is high in the adolescent boys of rural population. As regarding the awareness of biological symptoms related to HIV/AIDS in adolescent boys of urban area (31%) and rural area (28%). As well as awareness of treatment of HIV/AIDS in adolescent boys of urban area (40%) in rural area adolescent boys (32%) respectively. It is clear from Table – 2 that there is no statistical significant difference among the adolescent boys of urban area and rural area on their awareness of HIV/AIDS. The result of the present study show that belonging to rural localities both girls and boys adolescent have the lowest level of awareness regarding the transmission of HIV/AIDS which is very alarming stage. In rural area's adolescent girls and boys displayed less awareness of protection from the disease.

Table – 2 Distribution of adolescent boys according to their awareness regarding HIV/AIDS

Respondents (Boys)	average score	HIV/AIDS % average score	Awareness of				average score	mean score	S.D.	t
	Transmission	Misconception	Biological symptoms	Protection	Treatment					
Urban adolescents	33%	58%	31%	42%	40%	40.80	2.01	1.31	0.98
Rural adolescents	29%	61%	28%	30%	32%	36.00	1.89	1.6	

Although HIV/AIDS awareness is a problem of a society as a whole but it is more serious problem in the case of the adolescents. HIV/AIDS awareness is an unavoidable necessity for each and every individual especially for those who are in their teens/ adolescent period of age. Having knowledge about the various modes of transmission is a key factor for prevention of HIV/AIDS. HIV/AIDS awareness / education for adolescent and young people plays a vital role in global efforts to and the AIDS epidemic. Providing adolescent as well as young people with basic HIV/AIDS education enables them to protect themselves from becoming infected.

Acknowledgement:

The author of the present study gratefully acknowledges the cooperation of all the individuals who participated in the present study. As well as under thanks responsible entities which kindly helped in the present study.

REFERENCE

Bhan, N. B.Mahajan, P. Sondhi, M. (2004) Awareness regarding sex knowledge among Adolescent girls, Anthropologist, 6, (2), P. 101 -103.

Fantahum, M. & Chala, F. (1996) Sexual behavior and knowledge and attitude towards HIV/AIDS among out of school youth in baehi Dar Town, northwest Ethiopia Ethiopian Medical Journal, 34 (4) P. 233- 242

Ganguli, S. K., Pege, P., Gupta, N.,Charan, U. A. (2002) AIDS awareness among undergraduate students, Maharashtra, Indian Journal of Public Health, Vol. -46, (1) P. 8-12.

GuptaG.R.(2002) How Many power over women fuels the HIV epidemic ITS limits women's ability to contro sexual interactions British medical Jo 324 183-184.

Gregson S; Garmett G.P. Nyamukpa C.A. Hallet T. B. Lewis S. S. Cmason P. (2002) Anderson with behavior change in Eastern Zimbabure Science 311 (5761) 664-666.

Khurana, P. (2005) The awesome challenge of AIDS, Diamond Pocket Books, New Delhi.

MIC Manus, A, Dhar L (2008) Study of knowledge perception and attitude of adolescent girls tower STL/ HIV safer sex and education.BMC Women's Health Innovation Research Institute, Uni. Of Technology Perth, Australia.

Mahajan, P. & Sharma, N. (2005) Awareness level of Adolescent girls regarding HIV/AIDS (A comparative study of rural and urban area of Jammu), Journal of Human Ecol. 17, (4) p. 313 -314.

Momoh, S. O., Moses, A. L.and Ugiomoh, M. M. (2006) Women and the HIV/AIDS Epidemic, The Issue of School Age Girls Awareness in Nigeria, Journal of International Women Studies 8(1) P. 212.

National AIDS Control Organization (NACO) (1998-99) Country scenario NACO Ministry of health and Family welfare, Government of India, New Delhi.

Pavri, Khorshed M. (2005) Challenges of AIDS, National book Trust, New Delhi.

Payal Mahajan and Neeru Sharma (2005) Awareness level of adolescents girls regarding HIV/AIDS, Journal of Human Ecology, 17 (4) P. 313-314.

Pradhan, K. & Ramamani (2006) Gender impact on HIV/AIDS in India, New Delhi.

SARI Fact Sheet (2012) The Link between Sexual Violence and HIV.

UNA IDS (2000) Report on the global HIV/AIDS epidemic, June Geneva UNAIDS.

UNAIDS (2013) Global Report; UNAIDS report on the Global AIDS epidemic Geneva Switzerland.

United Nations Program me (2006) Gender impact on HIV/AIDS in India.

HIV/AIDS and Sex Workers in India

Ajay Chauhan[20]

ABSTRACT

AIDS is the advanced stage of HIV infection. It is disabling and incurable infection caused by HIV. As HIV progressively destroys the immune system, most people, particularly in resource constrained settings, die within a few years of the appearance of the first sighs of AIDS. Only a blood test can establish a person's HIV status. However, this does not mean that every person who undergoes the test has AIDS. Sex workers form a diverse group of people. Hence, it is difficult to make generalizations about their behaviors and attitudes towards HIV prevention and care.

Keywords: *HIV/AIDS, Sex Worker, India*

HIV is the acronym for human immunodeficiency virus. A person infected with HIV is medically known as an HIV-positive person.

AIDS stands for acquired immune deficiency syndrome.
- 'Acquired' means neither innate nor inherited, but transmitted from one infected
- person to another
- 'Immune' is the body's system of defence
- 'Deficiency' means not functioning to the appropriate degree
- 'Syndrome' means a group of signs and symptoms

AIDS is the advanced stage of HIV infection. It is a disabling and incurable infection caused by HIV. As HIV progressively destroys the immune system, most people, particularly in resource-constrained settings, die within a few years of the appearance of the first signs of AIDS. Only a blood test can establish a person's HIV

---

[20] M.Phil, Clinical Psychology, Sardar Patel University

status. However, this does not mean that every person who undergoes the test has AIDS. In healthy individuals, infections are kept away by a variety of defenders in the body. These defenders constitute the immune system of our body. Unknown to us, the immune system is at work every day, recognizing foreign bodies (e.g. bacteria, virus, etc.) and fighting them by producing specific chemicals called antibodies which neutralize foreign bodies. Each disease stimulates the production of antibodies specific to it. The detection of these antibodies in blood samples is therefore used to determine past or present infection. Since HIV causes damage to the immune system, the body cannot be protected against other infections, some of which then become the direct cause of death.

The Government of India estimates that about 2.40 million Indians are living with HIV (1.93 -3.04 million) with an adult prevalence of 0.31% (2009). Children (<15 yrs) account for 3.5% of all infections, while 83% are the in age group 15-49 years. Of all HIV infections, 39% (930,000) are among women. India's highly heterogeneous epidemic is largely concentrated in only a few states — in the industrialized south and west, and in the north-east. The four high prevalence states of South India (Andhra Pradesh – 500,000, Maharashtra – 420,000, Karnataka – 250,000, Tamil Nadu – 150,000) account for 55% of all HIV infections in the country. West Bengal, Gujarat, Bihar and Uttar Pradesh are estimated to have more than 100,000 PLHA each and together account for another 22% of HIV infections in India.

The Indian epidemic is concentrated among vulnerable populations at high risk for HIV. The concentrated epidemics are driven by unprotected sex between sex workers and their clients and by injecting drug use with contaminated injecting equipment. Several of the most at risk groups have high and still rising HIV prevalence rates. According to India's National AIDS Control Organization (NACO), the bulk of HIV infections in India occur during unprotected heterosexual intercourse. Consequently, and as the epidemic has matured, women account for a growing proportion of people living with HIV, especially in rural areas. The low rate of multiple partner concurrent sexual relationships among the wider community seems to have, so far, protected the larger body of people. However, although overall prevalence remains low, even relatively minor increases in HIV infection rates in a country of more than one billion people translate into large numbers of people becoming infected

Recent data suggests there are signs of a decline in HIV prevalence among female sex workers in areas where focused interventions have been implemented, particularly in the southern states, although overall prevalence levels among other high risk group continues to be high. The HIV prevalence as per HSS 2010 are: female sex workers 2.61%; men having sex with men 5.01%; injecting drug users 5.91 %; and transgender 18.80 %

HIV stands for human immunodeficiency virus. If left untreated, HIV can lead to the disease AIDS (acquired immunodeficiency syndrome).

Unlike some other viruses, the human body cannot get rid of HIV. That means that once you have HIV, you have it for life. No safe and effective cure for HIV currently exists, but scientists are working hard to find one, and remain hopeful.

HIV affects specific cells of the immune system, called CD4 cells, or T cells. Over time, if left untreated, HIV can destroy so many of these cells that the body can't fight off infections and disease. However, with proper medical care, HIV can be controlled. Treatment for HIV is called antiretroviral therapy or ART. It involves taking a combination of HIV medicines (called an HIV regimen) every day. Today, a person who diagnosed with HIV before the disease is far advanced and who gets and stays on ART can live a nearly normal life span.

The only way to know for sure if you have HIV is to get tested. Testing is relatively simple. You can ask your health care provider for an HIV test. Many medical clinics, substance abuse programs, community health centers, and hospitals offer them, too. You can also get an FDA-approved home HIV testing kit (the Home Access HIV-1 Test System or the OraQuick In-Home HIV Test) from a drugstore

Where Did HIV Come From?
Scientists identified a type of chimpanzee in West Africa as the source of HIV infection in humans. They believe that the chimpanzee version of the immunodeficiency virus (called simian immunodeficiency virus, or SIV) most likely was transmitted to humans and mutated into HIV1800s. Over decades, the virus slowly spread across Africa and later into other parts of the world. We know that the virus has existed in the United States since at least the mid- to late 1970s.

WHO ARE SEX WORKERS?
Sex workers form a diverse group of people. Hence, it is difficult to make generalizations about their behaviours and attitudes towards HIV prevention and care. For example, they may be IDUs, married women or men, indentured workers (i.e. people coerced into sex work and even taken to other countries), college students, unattached minors and may belong to any gender (i.e. male, female or transgender). They may work temporarily as sex workers or be full-time sex workers.

Sex workers have particular needs, and VCT and psychosocial interventions should be tailored specifically to these to ensure effectiveness. It is crucial that VCT services reach this vulnerable population; both to protect sex workers from HIV and other STIs, and to prevent transmission to their clients and partners. There is increasing evidence that targeted programmers to reduce the transmission of HIV infection within core groups are feasible and effective, and have led to successful risk reduction and decreased levels of infection.

Effective VCT interventions need to recognize sex workers not only as sex workers but also recognize the other dimensions of their lives as partners, wives or husbands, and as parents. There are different types of sex workers—street-based, lodge-based, brothel-based, community and caste-based, and even family-based. For most, sex work is a means of part-time livelihood. Most sex workers are young and married, and live with their husbands and children

HIV AND SEX WORKERS IN INDIA:

Number of female sex workers: 868,000
HIV prevalence: 2.7 percent
HIV prevention activities coverage: 84.5 percent

HIV prevalence among female sex workers varies both between and within states. For example, one study found HIV prevalence among sex workers ranged between 2 percent and 38 percent (averaging at 14.5 percent) among districts in the four high prevalence south Indian states such as, Andhra Pradesh, Maharashtra, Tamil Nadu and Karnataka.

Although sex work is not strictly illegal in India, associated activities - such as running a brothel – are. This means that the authorities can justify police hostility and brothel raids. Stigma and discrimination against sex workers restrict their access to healthcare.

Male sex workers are a group particularly vulnerable to HIV who engages in high-risk behaviours. One study in suburban Mumbai reported an HIV prevalence of 33 percent among this group with all of the individuals in the study engaging in anal sex while 13 percent had never used a condom.

When humans hunted these chimpanzees for meat and came into contact with their infected blood. Studies show that HIV may have jumped from apes to humans as far back as the late Hiv and sex workers:

Sex work is defined as the use of sexual activity for income or employment or for non-monetary items, such as food, drugs, or shelter ("survival" sex). Sex work can increase a person's risk of becoming infected with or transmitting HIV and other sexually transmitted infections (STIs) by engaging in unsafe sexual behaviors and/or substance use.

Sex work crosses many socioeconomic groups. Adults who engage in such activities include high-end escorts; people who work in massage parlors and the adult film industry; exotic dancers; state-regulated prostitutes (in Nevada); and street-based men, women, and transgender people who participate in survival sex.

Reaching sex workers is a critical effort for public health. Not only are sex workers at risk for higher rates of HIV and other STIs, sex workers who are unaware of their HIV status can endanger their own health and increase their risk of transmitting HIV or STIs to others

.

In India, HIV seroprevalence rates among sex workers have ranged from 50–90% in Bombay, Delhi, and Chennai. However, HIV rates of only 10% have been observed among sex workers in Calcutta, a city on the drug route into the heart of India and one of the most impoverished urban areas in the world. Condom use has risen in Calcutta in recent years, from 3% in 1992 to 90% in 1999, compared with steady rates of low condom use among sex workers in other cities in India.

Pathways into sex work in India are 3-fold. First, many women are born into sex work as the family profession. The stigma associated with sex work, often coupled with residual caste system discrimination, severely limits educational and alternative economic opportunities. Second, many young women from rural areas and neighboring countries (e.g., Nepal, Bangladesh) are deceived, sold, or otherwise trafficked into sex work against their will. Driven by the extreme poverty facing their families and the lure of relatively large incomes, some women choose to return to sex work, albeit in a less coercive context, once they are returned to their homes. Sex workers in Calcutta are conservatively estimated to earn an hourly wage almost twice that of women in urban India Finally, some women, given limited options, choose sex work as a means to support their families after being widowed, divorced, or abandoned by their husbands. About 9% of a random sample of sex workers in the Sonagachi "red light" area stated that they entered the profession voluntarily. While some sex workers are street-based, the majority work, and often live, in brothels clustered in red light areas of big cities and small towns.

Effective HIV prevention programs among sex workers have been implemented in Brazil, Thailand, and Zaire. Community participation among sex workers in HIV prevention, however, is not guaranteed, as in the demise of a community-based HIV prevention program among sex workers in southern India.

REFERENCES:

A, Patel (2015), SOME CASE STUDIES OF AIDS PATIENTS, Amazon, Inc, USA, ISBN: 978-1-4943-5907-2, 2013 (First Edition), Page: 30

Asthana S, Oostvogels R. Community participation in HIV prevention: problems and prospects for community-based strategies among female sex workers in Madras. Soc Sci Med. 1996;43:133–148.

NACO (2013) 'Annual Report 2012-13, http://www.naco.gov.in, Retrieved 10:16, Aug 01, 2015, from http://www.naco.gov.in/upload/Publication/Annual%20Report/Annual%20 report%202012-13_English.pdf [1]

Panos Institute . The Hidden Cost of AIDS: The Challenge of HIV to Development. The Panos Institute; London: 1992.

Pegacao Brazil: sex and self-worth. AIDS Action. 1991;15:5.

Rao V, Gupta I, Lokshin M, et al. Sex workers and the cost of safe sex: the compensating differential for condom use among Calcutta prostitutes. J Dev Econ. 2003;71:585–603.

Schoeof BG. AIDS action-research with women in Kinshasa, Zaire. Soc Sci Med. 1993;37:1401–1413.

UNAIDS (2013), 'India: HIV and AIDS estimates (2013), http://www.unaids.org, Retrieved 10:16, Aug 01, 2015

Webs:

http://www.worldbank.org/en/news/feature/2012/07/10/hiv-aids-india
https://www.aids.gov/hiv-aids-basics/hiv-aids-101/what-is-hiv-aids
http://www.ncbi.nlm.nih.gov/pmc/articles/PMC2826108/
http://www.cdc.gov/hiv/group/sexworkers.html

Psycho-Social Rehabilitation Outcomes among HIV-AIDS Patients during One Year Study

Haleema Khatoon[21], Fareed Aslam Minhas[22]

ABSTRACT

*Objective: The objective of this study was to examine the effect of psycho-social rehabilitation outcome on the psychological issues of HIV patients, during one year study. **Method:** This study was conducted at Institute of Psychiatry, Benazir Bhutto Hospital Rawalpindi. Sample was solely selected from injecting drug users (IDUs). It was both mixed method approach, based on pre and post testing. **Result:** Statistical analysis showed significant results and describe the marked reduction in psychological symptoms. **Conclusion:** Although symptoms of HIV-AIDS is difficult to revert but the associated psychological symptoms can be catered by strengthening the coping skills of the patient.*

Keywords: HIV-AIDS, Psychological Issues, Psycho-Social Rehabilitation, Pre-Post Assessment, Intravenous Drug Users (IV)

In Pakistan the number of heroin dependents is 860,000 and the injecting drug users are estimated to be 430,000. About 5%-10% of HIV infections are attributable to injecting drug use (Degenhardt & Hall, 2012).Pakistan is declared as an HIV epidemic country (UNODC Drug Report, 2013) and there is a high co-relation between injecting drug use and HIV which is apparent in various studies across the region. Estimates of the prevalence among people who inject drugs are over 40% in many parts of the world (Bulletin of WHO, 2011).Pakistan is one of the three countries in Asia that

---

[21] Clinical Psychologist & Research Associate at Institute of Psychiatry & WHO Collaborating Centre, Benazir Bhutto Hospital, Rawalpindi Pakistan
[22] Professor of Psychiatry, Head Institute of Psychiatry & WHO Collaborating Centre, Benazir Bhutto Hospital, Rawalpindi, Pakistan
*Corresponding Author

report an expanding HIV epidemic. The number of people that became newly infected with HIV was higher in 2012 than the number of new infections in 2011.The HIV epidemic in Pakistan is mainly driven by high risk injecting and sexual behaviors among people who inject drugs (PWID). It has been estimated that 85,000 people (range: 48,000 - 160,000) were living with HIV in 2012 (UNAIDS, 2013).

A report published by National AIDS Control Program (2008),confirms that the overall prevalence of HIV among 15-49 year olds is low at < 0.1% (range: < 0.1- 0.2 %) HIV prevalence among street based people who inject drugs (PWID) ranges from 3.3 % in Pak-Pattan to 53 % in Faisalabad (HIV/AIDS Surveillance Project, Round IV, GoP). In 2012 an estimated 19,000 people became newly infected with HIV in Pakistan (UNAIDS, 2013). According to a household survey supported by UNODC Pakistan Country Office in 2012 the annual prevalence of injection drug use among people aged 15 and 64 is 0.4% (range: 0.2% - 0.6%). This translates to approximately 430,000 people who inject drugs (range: 190,000 to 657,000).

Kumar (2002) reports 90% of worlds opium is being produced in Asia, and 60% of world opium users live in Asia, overall, however, there is a sub level of coverage in terms of treatment, outreach work, and provision of sterile needles and condoms, and provision in criminal justice system. A wealth of evidence exists globally about efficacy of specific interventions that prevent transmission of HIV among people who inject drugs. WHO, UNODC and UNAIDS recommend that all countries that report large scale use/injection of opiates should provide a comprehensive package of nine HIV prevention, treatment, and care interventions for PWID(WHO, 2012).

The other components of the package are Needle & Syringe exchange programs, HIV Testing and counseling, Anti-Retroviral therapy, Prevention and treatment of sexually transmitted diseases, Condom provision to patients and families, targeted information and education to IDUs, Diagnosis, vaccination and treatment of hepatitis B and Tuberculosis. To successfully address the treatment issue of HIV a comprehensive approach is required. Empirical evidence exists to demonstrate little impact of single interventions (Degenhardt et al., 2010).

Most patients with serious, progressive illness confront a range of psychological challenges, including the prospect of real and anticipated losses, worsening quality of life, the fear of physical decline and death, and coping with uncertainty. HIV infection and/or AIDS brings additional challenges duet other apidly changing treatment developments and outlook. In addition, this disease is unusual in the extent of stigma associated with it and the fact that HIV is both infectious and potentially fatal. Because of the risk of transmission, major and permanent changes are called for in sexual behavior and/or management of substance use, neither of which may be easily modifiable (Remien & Rabkin, 2001). Extensive research has been carried out within the field of mental health on the effectiveness of different types of psychological interventions. There is a significant amount of evidence around the effectiveness of cognitive behavioral interventions, mixed evidence for counselling, and lots of evidence for using motivational interviewing techniques in the substance misuse field (NAT, 2010).

METHOD

Sample: This study was conducted in the Institute of Psychiatry, Benazir Bhutto Hospital Rawalpindi. This is a 50 bedded Tertiary Care Facility, where was for the integration of psychiatry in the primary health care has been carried out and the site where mental health gap program has been launched and delivered in the 16 pilot districts of Pakistan. Sample was solely selected from injecting drug users which was filter at the drug detoxification and rehabilitation unit at the institute. A total of 121 IV drug users were identified and recruited from around the locality of Benazir Bhutto Hospital latterly, 31 HIV positive patients were selected. Following inclusion and exclusion criteria were used.

Inclusion criteria: a) Age more than 18 years b) Capable of giving Informed consent c) Drug users meeting ICD-10 [International Classification of Diseases-10] diagnosis for opioid dependence (as per self-report) at the time of interview with history of injecting drug use (ever use) and current users(last one month d) History of opioid dependence for a period of 5 years or longer. e) Client who can come for medicines every day) Persons willing to participate voluntarily and provide informed consent.

Exclusion criteria: a) Patients with serious medical conditions like acute respiratory failure, acute hepatic disease, delirium tremens and current dependence on alcoholb) Female patients who are pregnant or breast-feedingd) Presence of major psychiatric illness or physical illness due to which patient is unable to cooperate for interview e) Clients living in faraway areas unable to come every day.

Instrument/Measure
1. ADDICTION SEVERITY INDEX- ASI

The Addiction Severity Index is a relatively brief, semi-structured interview designed to provide important information about aspects of a patient's life which may contribute to his/her substance abuse syndrome. It includes the following domains: Medical, Employment/Support, Alcohol, Drug, Legal, Family/Social, and Psychiatric. These domains will be used by the patient to answer subjective questions in each problem area and will be presented for reference at this point in the interview. It's a 5 point (0-4) scale for patients to rate the severity of their problems and the extent to which they feel treatment for them is important. 0 - Not at all 1 - Slightly 2 - Moderately 3 - Considerably 4 – Extremely. For the purpose of this interview, severity will be defined as need for treatment where there currently is none; or for an additional form or type of treatment where the patient is currently receiving some form of treatment. These ratings should be based upon reports of amount, duration, and intensity of symptoms within a problem area. The following is a general guideline for the ratings: 0-1 No real problem, treatment not indicated 2-3 Slight problem, treatment probably not necessary 4-5 Moderate problem, some treatment indicated 6-7 Considerable problem, treatment necessary 8-9 Extreme problem, treatment absolutely necessary. It is important to note that these ratings are not intended as estimates of the patient's potential benefit from treatment, but rather the extent to which some form of effective intervention is needed, regardless of whether that treatment is available or even in existence.

Addiction Severity Index (ASI) was applied at each individual for 4 times with 3 months interval. It describes the severity of the addiction problem on 7 domains including medical, alcohol, drugs, employment, legal, family and psychological.

2. WORLD HEALTH ORGANIZATION-QUALITY OF LIFE (WHOQOL-HIV BREF)

According to the World Health Organization (WHO), the quality of life (QOL) of an individual is essentially defined as the subjective evaluation by such individuals of their own personal life embedded within the context of their culture and values (Hsiung et al., 2011). The WHOQOL-HIV BREF produces six domain scores. Whereas the WHOQOL-100 has four items to present each facet, the WHOQOL-HIV BREF has only one item. Included in these, there are two items that examine General quality of life: question 1 asks about an individual's overall perception of quality of life and question 2 asks about an individual's overall perception of his or her health. Hence there are 31 items, representing the 30 facets. Five of these facets are specific to HIV/AIDS. It is rated on a 5 point Likert scale where 1 indicates low, negative perceptions and 5 indicates high, positive perceptions. Domain scores are calculated as per the guidelines given in the WHOQOL-HIV-BREF manual (WHO, 2002).

Procedure: It was both mixed method approach, Comparative study for quantitative analysis, cognitive studies and subjective assessment by the mental health professional and focus group discussion (qualitative data). Clients were identified and screened according to inclusion and exclusion criteria in out-patient department in main OPD, using a semi structured interview and Assist Scale. Eligible clients selected for the study were sent to the Drug Detoxification and Rehabilitation Centre earmarked for medical and psychiatric management. Then they were registered on the front desk and sent to the psychologist room. Each patient was assessed in a structured way using an input proforma and using Addiction Severity Index scale. Each patient was also assessed for motivation and booked for further evaluation for quality of life questionnaire. If all inclusion criteria were satisfied and the client gave his informed consent he was inducted in the study. From the psychologist room he was sent to the medical Doctor who would screen him according to a structured proforma especially developed for screening out any medical problems. If any co morbid illnesses were screened appropriate referrals were made. He was also referred to the laboratory for HIV testing. Recruited patients were then incorporated in to the rehabilitation program, we have structured a proper session room where the rehabilitation sessions take place. This program includes counselling, motivational interviewing, physical exercise, breathing exercise and progressive muscle relaxation exercises.

RESULT

Quantitative Analysis

Data was then analyzed using a software SPSS-14.0. Appropriate statistical tests were applied to find out the significance of the findings. Analysis of variance was also used to test the difference between the results at different point of time.

Data analysis based on age range indicates that most of the participants of the study were from the age range of 26-35 years (37%) there was also high level of addiction present in adulthood which is 46-65 years (23%). Our data analysis supports this argument that drug taking behavior is more common in late adolescence to adulthood. Since these are chronic dependent users who have had long history of drug taking behavior and numerous treatments and relapses many patients come into the category of 46-65. Based on the demographic data, it revealed that most of the participants were male (99%) female ratio was very low (1%). Percentage of unmarried people is high (48%) as compared to married people (35%) hence there is low ratio of participants who are either divorced/separated or widow/er. There was low percentage (18%) of participants who get high education rest of the participants were under metric (range 25-30%). Descriptive data also revealed that high frequency of the participants was unemployed (52%) but there was high ratio of the people who are skilled (68%).

Table 1: t-Test, Mean scores for overall quality of life and general health perceptions for six domains of WHOQOL-HIV BREF (N= 30).

Facets	Mean(±SD) Pre-Test	Mean(±SD) Post-Test	t	p
Physical Domain	17.0 (10.0)	22.6 (15.0)	-16.6	.000
Psychological Domain	14.0 (12.0)	28.6 (18.0)	-11.8	.000
Level of	14.4 (11.4)	23.5 (14.0)	-12.4	.000

independence Domain				
Social relationships Domain	12.3 (13.0)	22.5 (15.0)	-9.5	.000
Environment Domain	12.0 (13.0)	22.5 (14.6)	-9.2	.000
Spirituality/Religion/ personal belief Domain	19.0 (9.3)	23.3 (13.9)	-19.8	.000

Table 1 explains the results of six different domains of WHOQOL-HIV BREF. In physical domain at the pretest level mean score was 17 while at posttest level, mean score was 22.6. In psychological domain the mean score were 14.0 while at the post test level the mean score were 28.6. In the third domain i.e. level of independence mean score were 14.4 at the pretest level and at the post test level mean score were 23.5. In the social relationship domain at the pretest level mean score were 12.3 and at the post test level mean score were 22.5. In the environment domain mean score were 12.0 at the pretest level and 22.5 mean score were at the post test level. In the last domain spirituality/religion/ personal belief domain at the pretest level score were 19.0 and at the post test level the score were 23.3. Increase in mean score indicates better quality of life and it is evident from the results that the quality of life of the participants has improved during the period of pre and post testing

Figure 1: Pre and post assessment of WHOQOL-HIV BREF scores

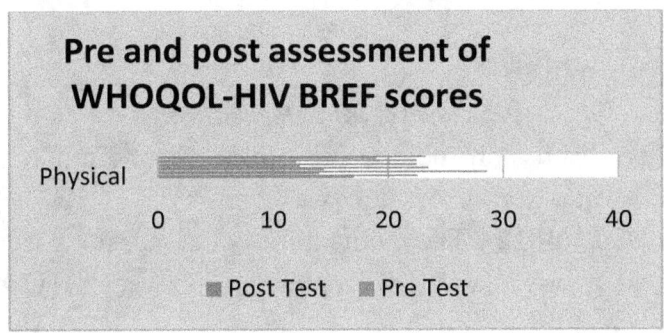

In the above figure mean scores of the 6 domains of WHOQOL-HIV BREF are showed at the pretest and posttest level. The above chart explains how quality of life of individuals has changed during the pretest and posttest level. Deviation in the post test level shows better quality of life in the participants.

Table 2: Cronbach's Alpha reliability of WHO-QOL-BREF (N= 30)

Scale		α*	No. of Domains
WHOQOL-HIV BREF	Baseline (Pre Test)	.99	6
	6 Month	.99	6
	9 Month	.99	6
	12 Month (Post Test)	.99	6

Note. *Cronbach's Alpha (Cronbach's alpha simply provides you with an overall reliability coefficient for a set of variables (e.g., questions).

Reliability analysis was done to check the appropriateness of the scale (i.e. WHO QOL-HIV BREF) for use with the targeted population. Data analysis explains that the cornbach's alpha is lies in the category of "excellent range (High-Stakes testing)" for this particular scale.

Qualitative Analysis
1.1 Focus Group on Psychosocial Intervention
Focus group discussion method utilized to get the qualitative data. The target group for discussion was consisted of HIV +ve male clients on OST (N=12). The main themes of discussions were related to awareness about HIV/AIDS, connection between HIV/AIDS and

drug abuse, change in life after diagnoses of HIV/AIDS, including stigma and role of psycho-social rehabilitation.

It was noted that almost all of the participants were well aware of HIV/AIDS and the risks behavior associated to it. Some of them got to know about it through media and NGOs while others got to know about it when they started drug treatment and got screened for Hep-C, B & HIV.

The general consensus was that there was a link between drug use, risky sexual behavior and HIV/AIDS. There was a high tendency for persons to share needles and engage in risky sexual behavior when under the influence of drugs since drug use altered one's ability to think. It was also noted that people got into injecting drug abuse initially on experimental basis or easy availability of syringes on the drugs hotspots and due to the peer pressure.

It was further noted that families of HIV+ve patients have showed different reactions when came to know about their loved ones' positive status. Some families became cooperative, some stigmatized and thrown them out of home and some were in denial that such epidemic could happen to their loved one.

It was also stated that HIV/AIDS has brought change in personalities of infected persons. Some became more careful about themselves and others, while some became careless towards life.
The treatment adherence and great satisfaction with the psycho-social rehabilitation was also noted among the participants as they don't have to take any illicit drug after taking OST daily dose. They remain active and free from opioid's withdrawals and craving.

As far as the treatment of HIV/AIDS concerned, it was noted that most of the clients with positive status have not started ART because some have low CD 4 count, some have poor financial status and lack of awareness related to HIV/AIDS treatment.

1.2 Quality of Life

The patient satisfaction & dissatisfaction reported on experience and reflecting QOL scores indicated that satisfaction can be defined as the extent of an individual's experience compared with his or her expectations. Patients' satisfaction is related to the extent to which general health care needs and condition-specific needs are met. Evaluating to what extent patients are satisfied with health services is clinically relevant, as satisfied patients are more likely to comply with treatment, take an active role in their own care, continue using medical care services, and stay with a particular health provider.

When Quality of Life questionnaire was administered at the baseline, a majority of clients reported to be highly dissatisfied with their lives. They were unemployed and social and occupational functioning was markedly impaired due to drug abuse. Their personal relationships, household and broader social functioning was also significantly impaired and in most cases the clients did not enjoy the support of their families. This was reflected by the QOL scores which indicated that their quality of life in all domains i.e. psychological, physical, spiritual, environment, level of independence and social relationships was poor. As reported by themselves as well as their families, mostly the clients spent their time in drug use and did not engage in productive or goal oriented activities.

When QOL was administered at different phases, significant improvements were seen in terms of QOL scores. When the questionnaire was administered at 12 months, majority of clients were found to have an improved quality of life. There were significant improvements in all domains especially psychological, social relationships and psychological. One aspect that was clearly identified was an improvement in occupational functioning as most of the clients were jobless at the time of induction but at 12 months were doing different jobs and earning for their families. This helped them to improve their personal relationships with their families and their self-confidence improved which was negligible at the beginning of the study. In keeping with the current evidence base which indicates that improvement in quality of life leads to improved compliance.

DISCUSSION

This study had a pre and post intervention design with assessments made at baseline and at three, six, nine and twelve months. A total of 210 subjects were recruited in the study, however those that were inducted in the study were 121. The study was conducted from January to December, 2013. The assessments were conducted using standard instruments and semi structured interviews. Interventions included medical treatment, motivational work, focus groups discussions, counselling and family work. WHO Quality of Life questionnaire was also applied. Laboratory investigations and referrals for management of respective problems was also an integral part of the study.

There is strong evidence that there is higher prevalence of mental health problems amongst people living with HIV compared with the general population. People with a mental health problem are at greater risk of HIV infection, and people who have been diagnosed with HIV are more likely to develop a mental health problem, for example anxiety or depression.

Psychiatric management of HIV-infected individuals
Specific techniques that establish the psychiatric management of patients with HIV/AIDS include the following 1) establishing and maintaining a therapeutic alliance 2) collaboration and coordination of care with other mental health and medical providers 3) diagnosing

and treating all associated psychiatric disorders 4) facilitating adherence to the overall treatment plan 5) providing education about psychological, psychiatric, and neuropsychiatric disorders 6) providing risk reduction strategies to further minimize the spread of HIV; maximizing psychological and social/ adaptive functioning 7) considering the role of religion/spirituality 8) preparing the patient for issues of disability, death, and dying 9)and advising family regarding sources of care and support. The development of a psychiatric treatment plan for patients with HIV infection requires thoughtful and comprehensive consideration of the biopsychosocial context of the illness (Science, 1996).

CONCLUSION

When seeing a patient in consultation, it is important to gather history about cognitive or motor symptoms and conduct a mental status screening examination to determine whether neurocognitive deficits are present. Psychiatrists should be knowledgeable about medication side effects and drug interactions of psychotropic agents as well as HIV-related medications in order to provide optimum patient care. Psychiatric treatment of patients with HIV infection should include active monitoring of substance abuse, since it is often associated with risk behaviors that can lead to further transmission of HIV. Adherence is of utmost concern with antiretroviral treatment because the regimens are so unforgiving; even minor deviations from the prescribed regimen can result in viral resistance and permanent loss of efficacy for existing medications. Psychiatrists can play an important role in the promotion of patient adherence, since comorbid psychiatric disorders (e.g., substance abuse or depression) have been shown to adversely affect patient compliance with a complicated treatment regimen.

ACKNOWLEDGEMENTS

We acknowledge UNAIDS, UNODC and WHO as part of a comprehensive package of nine core interventions for IDU programs that collectively maximize impact for HIV prevention and treatment.

DECLARATION OF INTEREST & FUNDING

The author declares no potential conflicts of interest with respect to the authorship and/or publication of this article and there is no funding involved in this research project by any organization.

REFERENCES

Bulletin of the World Health Organization. (2011). 89 (10), 701-701. doi:10.2471/BLT.11.001011

Degenhardt, L., Mathers, B., &Guarinieri, M., et al. (2010). Meth/amphetamine use and associated HIV: implications for global policy and public health. *International Journal of Drug Policy, 21,* 347-358.

Degenhardt, L.,& Hall, W. (2012). Extent of illicit drug use and dependence, and their contribution to the global burden of disease. *The Lancet,379*(9810), 55-70.

Hsiung, P. C. 1., Fang, C. T., Wu, C. H., Sheng, W. H., Chen, S. C., Wang, J. D., Yao, G. (2011). Validation of the WHOQOL-HIV BREF among HIV-infected patients in Taiwan.*AIDS Care, 23*(8), 1035-42. doi: 10.1080/09540121.2010.543881.

Kumar, M. S. (2002). HIV Prevention Strategies for Injection Drug Users in High HIV-Prevalent Scenarios. Global Research Network on HIV Prevention in Drug-Using Populations.Fourth Annual Meeting. National Institute of Health. United States Department of Health and Human Services.

National AIDS Control Program, Ministry of Health, Government of Pakistan. HIV/AIDS Surveillance Project 2004-2008. http://www.nacp.gov.pk/programme_partners/cida/

National AIDS Trust (NAT). July 2010. Psychological support services for people living with HIV.

Robert, H. R., & Judith G. R. (2001). Psychological aspects of living with HIV disease. A primary care perspective. *West J Med, 175,*332-335.

UNAIDS report on the global AIDS epidemic. (2013). GLOBAL REPORT. Retrieved from http://www.unaids.org/sites/default/files/media_asset/UNAIDS_Glo bal_Report_2013_en_1.pdf

United Nation Organization on Drugs and Crime report. Drug use in Pakistan, 2013. Retrieved from https://www.unodc.org/documents/pakistan/Survey_Report_Final_ 2013.pdf

WHO, UNODC, UNAIDS. (2012). Technical Guide for countries to set targets for universal access to HIV prevention, treatment and care for injecting drug users.

World Health Organization (2002). Department of Mental Health and Substance Dependence World Health Organization. Geneva: Switzerland. Retieved from http://www.who.int/mental_health/media/en/613.pdf

Mindfulness Based Cognitive Therapy for Depression among HIV- Infected Individuals

Baijesh A. R.[23]

ABSTRACT

People living with HIV/AIDS are at a higher risk for depression and mostly goes both undiagnosed and untreated. Untreated depression is a grave concern, researches indicate that it can lead to significant distress, functional impairment and can cause psychological suffering along with worse medical outcomes, including immunosuppressive effects. Antiretroviral Therapy (ART) is a widely used and promising treatment strategy for individuals infected with HIV. Studies indicate that treatment of clinical depression can enhance the treatment adherence to ART and recovery from depression is correlated with increased CD4 cell counts. The present study is a preliminary investigation, evaluating the efficacy of MBCT in the management of Depression among HIV infected individuals who are undergoing ART. A total of 10 individuals with HIV infection undergoing ART since 2-3 months who were also diagnosed with clinical depression in a community clinic were recruited for the study. There were 5 drop-outs, and the remaining 5 participants subjected to an 8 week MBCT treatment program for depression. The participants were assessed by Beck Depression Inventory- II (BDI) and Hospital Anxiety Depression Scale (HADS), pre- and post intervention. The assessment scores, pre- and post-intervention, were compared and was found as statistically significant at 0.05 level on both HADS Depression subscale (z= -2.07) and BDI (z=-2.02). Post- intervention, all 5 participants were interviewed by an independent clinician for depression, and only one person met the ICD-10 diagnostic criteria for depression. The findings of the study indicate a preliminary efficacy of MBCT in treating clinical depression among people infected with HIV.

---

[23] Central University of Karnataka
*Corresponding Author

Keywords: HIV-AIDS, Mindfulness Based Cognitive Therapy
(MBCT), ART

India has the third largest HIV epidemic in the world. The
prevalence of HIV in India was estimated as 0.3% in 2013. This
figure equates to 2.1 million people living with HIV (UNAIDS,
2014). It is also observed that, India's HIV epidemic is slowing
down, with a 19% decline in new HIV infections, and a 38% decline
in AIDS-related deaths between 2005 and 2013 (UNAIDS, 2014).
The prevalence of HIV in India varies geographically. The five
states with the highest HIV prevalence are Nagaland, Mizoram,
Manipur, Andhra Pradesh and Karnataka (NACO, 2014).

In India since the year 2004, free ART has been available. At ART
clinics, people living with HIV can access testing and counselling,
nutritional advice and treatment for HIV and opportunistic
infections. CD4 count test in every six months was made mandatory
for the patients (NACO, 2013). There are lots of promotional
activities to remind people about their testing appointments with the
aim of increasing overall attendance (WHO, 2013). However, in
2013, only 36% of adults eligible for ART received treatment,
alongside 30% of children (UNAIDS, 2014). The introduction of the
WHO (2013) treatment guidelines has increased the access to ART.

The two most prevalent and interfering psychosocial comorbidities
of HIV infection are clinical depression and substance use (Berger-
Greenstein et al., 2007; Bing et al., 2001; Ruiz Perez et al., 2005).
Clinical depression and problematic substance use not only can
cause significant distress and functional impairment, but also can
interfere with HIV treatment and care; both conditions have
consistently been associated with poor antiretroviral therapy (ART)
adherence (Catz, Kelly, Bogart, Benotsch, & McAuliffe, 2000;
DiMatteo, Lepper, & Croghan, 2000; Lucas, Cheever, Chaisson, &
Moore, 2001; Lucas, Gebo, Chaisson, & Moore, 2002; Paterson et
al., 2000; Safren et al., 2001).

People living with HIV/AIDS (PHA) not only experience depression
at high rates, also frequently goes both undiagnosed and untreated.
For PHA, untreated depression is a grave concern, as it can lead to

psychological suffering and worse medical outcomes, including immunosuppressive effects and death. Berger-Greenstein and colleagues (2007) reported that over 70% of participants met criteria for major depression among a sample of patients diagnosed with HIV, substance abuse, and psychiatric illness. In a randomized controlled trial among HIV-infected injection drug users during an evaluation of depressive symptoms and symptomatic response in a directly observed ART, improvements in depression over six months found as associated with increases in CD4 cell count and adherence, while worsening in depression was found associated with active drug use and increases in plasma viral RNA levels (Attia et al., 2009; Hull & Montaner, 2011; Springer, Chen, & Altice, 2009).

Mindfulness-Based Stress Reduction (MBSR) has been used to improve quality of life and enhance outcomes among many groups. Recent studies indicate that MBSR may enhance immune function in PHA. Mindfulness-Based Cognitive Therapy (MBCT), an 8-week skills-based group intervention, combines MBSR with Cognitive Therapy to prevent depressive relapse. There are number of research evidences suggesting that MBCT may be an effective means of treating depression (Hofmann, et al., 2010; Kuyken & Williams, 2012). Research studies showed that MBCT could reduce self reported distress, and improve quality of life and healthier HIV biomarkers, indicating its effectiveness for the psychological treatment of HIV/AIDS (Gonzalez- Gazia et al., 2013; Rodriguez, T., 2014).

METHOD

Aim

The aim of the present study is to evaluate the efficacy of MBCT in the management of Depression among HIV infected individuals who are undergoing ART.

Participants

The sample consisted of clients selected from the General Hospital who were diagnosed by a consultant psychiatrist and clinical psychologist as having mild or moderate depressive episodes according to the International Classification of Diseases-10 (ICD-10) criteria. Clients with

co-morbid psychiatric conditions were excluded from the study. 10 participants were recruited to the study as referred by the consultant Psychiatrist. Seven of the participants were males and three females. The mean age of the sample was 32.5 years (range = 24- 45 years) and the mean duration of illness was 6 years (range = 4-8 years). All ten participants were ART for HIV since last 2-3 months. Of the ten patients four were married and six were single. All the clients had formal education, and all were of middle socioeconomic status, living in a urban locality currently not working. The participants were not not under any psychiatrc medications for the mood problems.

Design

A single group pre-post test design was used in the study to examine the outcome of MBCT with regards to reducing symptoms of depression among HIV infected individuals. Figure 1 shows the study design.

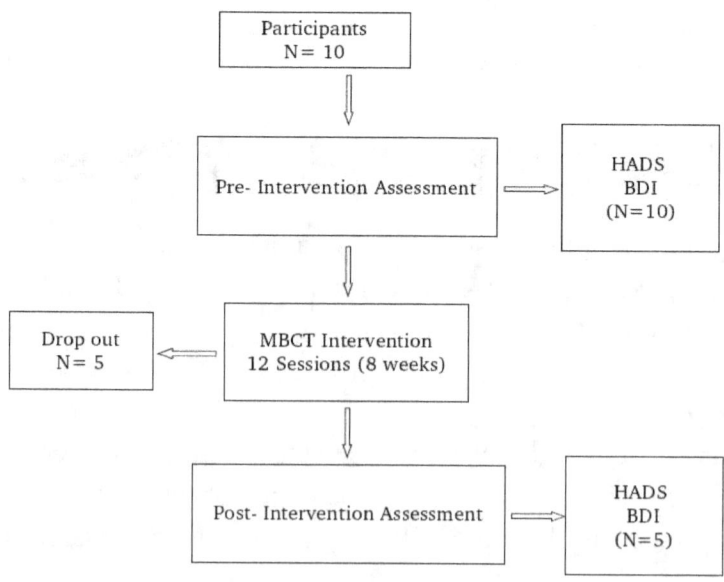

Tools

A Sociodemographic and Clinical Data Sheet was used to obtain information on the demographic and clinical history. The Hospital Anxiety Depression Scale (HADS) and Beck Depression Inventory-II (BDI) was used in quantifying Depression and anxiety experienced by the patient.

Procedure

The patients were assessed on HADS and BDI pre- & post-intervention a by an independent rater. Therapeutic program : The therapeutic program consisted of 8 sessions for each client over a period of eight weeks. The sessions were conducted individually, every treatment had the same format. Each session lasted for approximately 90-120 minutes. The treatment followed the Mindfulness Based Cognitive Therapy (MBCT) Implementation Resources by Kuyken et al., (2012).

Dropout: Though 10 individuals were recruited for the program, five of them did not complete the program due to various reasons. One person met with an accident and passed away, while three of them shifted to different cities for treatment and care. One person did not show up after the first session at all, discontinued ART as well.

Analysis

Statistical analysis was carried out on the five patients. The Wilcoxon signed-rank test was used to analyse the data. The pre-treatment HADS & BDI scores were compared with post-treatment scores to evaluate the outcome of MBCT intervention. For analyzing the data GNU PSPP statistical software version 0.7.9. was used.

Apart from that clinically significant changes (50% and above) based on pre- & post-therapy was used to assess the efficacy of the therapeutic intervention. The percentage of change between pre- and post-therapy points was calculated using the following Blanchard and Schwartz (1988) formula.

$$\frac{\text{Pre Score} - \text{Post Score}}{\text{Pre Score}} \times 100 = \text{Therapeutic Change}$$

And

$$\frac{\text{Pre Score} - \text{Follow-up Score}}{\text{Pre Score}} \times 100 = \text{Therapeutic Change}$$

RESULTS AND DISCUSSION

The aim of the present study was to evaluate the efficacy of MBCT in the management of Depression among HIV infected individuals who are undergoing ART.

Table 1 shows the pre- & post intervention assessment scores on HADS & BDI with improvement percentage for five patients who completed the treatment.

Table 1

Sl. No	HADS- D pre	HADS-D post	IP	HADS-A pre	HADS- A post	IP	BDI pre	BDI post	IP
1	13	6	53.84*	8	6	50*	24	10	58.33*
2	15	7	53.33*	10	6	40	28	12	57.14*
3	14	6	57.14*	5	5	0	22	11	50*
4	16	8	50*	9	3	66.67*	32	14	56.25*
5	16	9	43.75	11	5	54.55*	30	18	40

IP: improvement percentage (in %); * clinically significant ; HADS- D: Hospital Anxiety Depression Scale- Depression sub- scale; HADS- D: Hospital Anxiety Depression Scale- Anxiety subscale; BDI- Beck Depression Inventory- II.

The comparison of pre and post intervention mean scores on HADS-D , HADS- A & BDI scores using Wilcoxon Signed Rank Test is shown in Table 2.

Table 2

Measure	z	p
HADS -D	-2.07	0.04*
HADS- A	-1.84	0.07
BDI	-2.02	0.04*

HADS- D: Hospital Anxiety Depression Scale- Depression subscale;
HADS- D: Hospital Anxiety Depression Scale- Anxiety subscale;
BDI- Beck Depression Inventory- II; * : significant at 0.05 level

After completion of the intervention, clinical interview by the referred psychiatrist indicated significant improvement in four individuals and they did not meet the diagnostic criteria for depression anymore, where as one person still met with the diagnostic requirements for depression. The analysis of the results for individual cases suggests that on HADS-D, improvement was observed in the reported level of depression at the completion of intervention among all the clients, in which four participants showed clinically significant change on this measure. While on HADS-A, the improvement in scores was observed among only four in which three had a clinically significant improvement. While, on BDI, there was improvement in the reported depression levels of all five participants at post intervention while only four of them had clinically significant change.

Analysis of results on all three measures revealed that MBCT was effective in bringing about statistically significant reduction in depression among HIV infected individuals who was undergoing ART.

In conclusion, the findings of this investigation indicate that MBCT can be an effective intervention in the management of depression among HIV infected individuals. The findings are in consistent with the previous studies (Gonzalez- Gazia et al., 2013; Rodriguez, T., 2014) indicating the efficacy ob MBCT.

The study has some significant implications. This is the first study to be carried out in India, which has adopted MBCT in the management of HIV infected patients with Depression undergoing ART. The significant reduction in depressive symptoms that occurred in the patients following the intervention point towards the efficacy of MBCT.

The small sample size is a significant limitation of the present study, as it does not allow for rigorous analysis of data and generalization of results. The inclusion of a control group would have strengthened the study. The absence of a follow-up is another limitation, as it would provide information on the maintenance of treatment gains. Future research should be conducted with larger samples, longer follow-up and control groups to establish and generalize the efficacy of this program.

REFERENCES

Amico, K.R., Harman, J.J., & Johnson, B.T. (2006). Efficacy of antiretroviral therapy adherenceinterventions: A research synthesis of trials, 1996 to 2004. *Journal of Acquired Immune Deficiency Syndromes, 41,* 285-297.

Amir, L. (1997). HIV infection in pregnant women in South Australia. *Medical Journal of Australia, 166,* 470-472.

Bansberg, D.R. (2006). Less than 95% adherence to nonnucleoside reverse-transcriptase inhibitor therapy can lead to viral suppression. *Clinical Infectious Diseases, 43,* 942-944.

Bartlett J.A. (2002). Addressing the challenges of adherence. *Journal of Acquired Immune Deficiency Syndromes, 29*, S2-S10.

Centers for Disease Control and Prevention (CDC) (2006). Epidemiology of HIV/AIDS – United States, 1981-2005. *Morbidity and Mortality Weekly Report, 55*, 589-592.

Chiesa, A., & Serretti, A. (2011). Mindfulness based cognitive therapy for psychiatric disorders: Asystematic review and meta-analysis. *Psychiatry Review, 187*, 441–453.

Clark, D.M., Ball, S., & Pape, D. (1991). An experimental investigation of thought suppression,*Behaviour Research and Therapy, 29*, 253–257.

Coelho, H. F., Canter, P. H., & Ernst, E. (2007). Mindfulness-based cognitive therapy: Evaluating current evidence and informing future research. *Journal of Consulting and Clinical Psychology, 75*, 1000-1005.

Crum, N.F., Riffenburgh, R.H., Wegner, S., Agan, B.K., Tasker, S.A., Spooner, K.M., et al. (2006).Comparisons of causes of death and mortality rates among HIV- infected persons: analysis of thepre-, early, and late HAART (highly active antiretroviral therapy) eras. *Journal of Acquired Immune Deficiency Syndromes, 41*,194-200.

Forman, E.M., Butryn, M., Hoffman, K.L., & Herbert, J.D. (2009). An open trial of an acceptance-based behavioral treatment for weight loss. *Cognitive Behavioral Practice, 16*, 223-235.

Gonzalez- Garcia, M., Ferrer, M. J., Borras, X., Munoz- Moreno, J. A., Miranda, C., Puig, J. et al., (2013). Effectiveness of Mindfulness-Based Cognitive Therapy on the Quality of Life, Emotional Status, ans CD4 Cell Count of Patients Aging with HIV Infection. *AIDS and Behavior 18*(4), 676-685. Abstract retrieved from NCBI-PubMed database.

Hofmann, S. G., Sawyer, A. T., Witt, A. A., & Oh, D. (2010). The effect of mindfulness-based therapy on anxiety and depression: A meta-analytic review. *Journal of Consultant Clinical Psychology, 78*, 169-183.

Johnson, M.O., Charlebois, E., Morin, S.F., Catz, S.L., Goldstein, R.B., Remien, R.H., et al. (2005). Perceived adverse effects of antiretroviral therapy. *Journal of Pain Symptom Management, 29*, 193-205.

Jones, D.L., Ishii, M., LaPerriere, A., Stanley, H., Antoni, M., Ironson, G., et al. (2003). Influencing medication adherence among women with AIDS. *AIDS Care, 15*, 463-474.

Kuyken, W., Byford, S., Taylor, R. S., Watkins, E., Holden, E., White, K., ... Teasdale, J. D. (2008). Mindfulness-based cognitive therapy to prevent relapse in recurrent depression. *Journal of Consulting and Clinical Psychology, 76,* 966–978.

Kuyken, W., & Williams, M. (2012). Mindfulness-Based Cognitive Therapy (MBCT) Implementation Resources. Oxford University. Retrieved from http://mindfulnessteachersuk.org.uk/pdf/MBCTImplementationRes ources.pdf

Madru, N. (2003). Stigma and HIV: Does the Social Response Affect the Natural Course of the Epidemic? *Journal of the Association of Nurses in AIDS care, 14,* 39-48.

Malcolm, S.E., Ng, J.J., Rosen, R.K., & Stone, V.E. (2003). An examination of HIV/AIDS patients who have excellent adherence to HAART. *AIDS Care, 15,* 251-261.

Mocroft, A., Ledergerber, B., Katlama, C., Kirk, O., Reiss, P., d'Arminio, M.A., et al. (2003). Decline in the AIDS and death rates in the EuroSIDA study: an observational study. *Lancet, 362,* 22-29.

NACO. (2014). Annual Report 2013-14. Retrieved from http://www.naco.gov.in/upload/2014%20mslns/NACO_English%2 02013-14.pdf

Paterson, D.L., Swindells, S., Mohr, J., Brester, M., Vergis, E.N., Squier, C., et al. (2000). Adherence to protease inhibitor therapy and outcomes in patients with HIV infection. *Annals of Internal Medicine, 133,* 21–30.

Rodriguez, T. (2014). The Role of Acceptance and Mindfulness in People Living With HIV/AIDs: A Meta-Analysis. (Electronic Thesis or Dissertation). Retrieved from https://etd.ohiolink.edu/!etd.send_file?accession=bgsu1404401086 &disposition=inline

SAMHSA's National Registry of Evidence-based Programs and practices. (2012). Mindfulness-Based Cognitive Therapy An Informational Resource. Comparative Effectiveness Research Series. Retrieved from http://www.nrepp.samhsa.gov/pdfs/MBCT_Booklet_Final.pdf

Schuster, M.A., Collins, R., Cunningham, W.E., Morton, S.C., Zierler, S., Wong, M., et al. (2005).Perceived discrimination in clinical care in a nationally representative sample of HIV-infected adults receiving health care. *Journal of General Internal Medicine, 20,* 807-813.

Segal, Z. V., Williams, J. M. G., & Teasdale, J. D. (2002). Mindfulness-based cognitive therapy fordepression: A new approach to preventing relapse. New York: The Guilford Press.

Simoni, J.M., Pearson, C.R., Pantalone, D.W., Marks, G., & Crepaz, N. (2006). Efficacy of interventions in improving highly active antiretroviral therapy adherence and HIV-1 RNA viral load: A meta- analytic review of randomized controlled trials. *Journal of Acquired Immune Deficiency Syndromes, 43*, S23-S35.

Taylor, S.E., Kemeny, M.E., Reed, G.M., Bower, J.E., & Gruenewald, T.L. (2000). Psychological Resources, Positive Illusions, and Health. *American Psychologist,55*, 99-109.

The Gap Report (2014). UNAIDS. Retrieved from http://www.unaids.org/sites/default/files/en/media/unaids/contenta ssets/documents/unaidspublication/2014/UNAIDS_Gap_report_en .pdf

Thompson, R.J., Gil, K.M., Abrams, M.R., & Phillips, G. (1992). Stress, coping, and psychological adjustment of adults with sickle cell disease. *Journal of Consulting and Clinical Psychology, 60*, 433-440.

Weaver, K.E., Llabre, M.M., Duran, R.E., Antoni, M.H., Ironson, G., Penedo, F.J., et al. (2005). A stress and coping model of medication adherence and viral load in HIV positive men and women on highly active antiretroviral therapy (HAART). *Health Psychology, 24*, 385-392.

WHO. (2013). Consolidated guidelines on the use of antiretroviral drugs for treating and preventing HIV infection. Retrived from http://www.who.int/hiv/pub/guidelines/arv2013/download/en/

WHO. (2013). Global update on HIV treatment 2013: Results, impact and opportunities. Retrieved from http://apps.who.int/iris/bitstream/10665/85326/1/9789241505734_eng.pdf

Psychotherapy in HIV/AIDS

Preeti Sharma[24], Mustafa Nadeem Kirmani[25]*

ABSTRACT

HIV/AIDS is a condition in which the immune system of the patient gets impaired and does not function properly so that the opportunistic infections occur in them which often causes mortality. It is caused by a retro virus which gets transferred through unprotected sexual intercourse with the person having the virus, through intravenous drug use, infected blood transfusion and other similar methods. Being infected with HIV is traumatic for the patient because the treatment of this disease is still in infancy they have to face lots of challenges in the treatment process. It creates an emotional and financial turmoil not just for the patient but for the whole family. Empirical and clinical work has shown that patients with HIV/AIDS experience lots of emotional and psychiatric issues. In India, these issues are often not focused by the treating physicians. However, recently these areas are being targeted and emotional and related issues faced by these patients have become the focus of interventions by the treating team. The current paper will focus on the various psychological issues faced by HIV/AIDS patients and psychological interventions which can be used to work on these issues. Since HIV/AIDS causes multitude of medical, psychological, social, economic and spiritual issues in the patients, holistic and biopsychsocio spiritual model of intervention need to be followed for better recovery and quality of life of these patients.

Keywords: HIV-AIDS, Psychotherapy

The first clinical cases of acquired immunodeficiency syndrome (AIDS) were identified in 1981. The human immunodeficiency virus

[24] Research Scholar, Department of Psychology, Pacific University, Udaipur, Rajasthan
[25] Doctorate Student, Department of Psychology, Aligarh Muslim University, Aligarh, UP
*Corresponding Author

(HIV), the causative agent of AIDS, was discovered in 1983. It is estimated that almost two million Americans have acquired HIV infection. Although AIDS was initially diagnosed in the United States in a group of gay men, groups recognized as at high risk for infection in this country include a wider sector of the population -- intravenous drug abusers (IVDAs), haemophiliacs and heterosexuals who have sex with patients belonging to high risk groups.). In 1983 an infectious agent, the Human immunodeficiency virus (HIV) was identified as the cause of AIDS. Since then world0 wide more than 7 million people have been diagnosed with AIDS, 4.5 million have died from HIV associated conditions, and probably around 21 million have been infected with HIV.

India has the third highest number of estimated people living with HIV in the world. India has a population of one billion, around half of whom are adults in the sexually active age group. The first AIDS case in India was detected in 1986 and since then HIV infection has been reported in all states and union territories. The spread of HIV in India has been uneven. Although much of India has a low rate of infection, certain places have been more affected than others. HIV epidemics are more severe in the southern half of the country and the far north-east. The highest HIV prevalence rates are found in Andhra Pradesh, Maharashtra, Tamil Nadu and Karnataka in the south; and Manipur and Nagaland in the north-east. In the southern states, HIV is primarily spread through heterosexual contact. Infections in the north-east are mainly found amongst injecting drug users (IDUs) and sex workers. (National AIDS Control Organisation, 2008).According to the HIV Estimations 2012, the estimated number of people living with HIV/AIDS in India was 20.89 lakh, with an estimated adult (15-49 age group) HIV prevalence of 0.27% in 2011. India has demonstrated an overall reduction of 57% in the annual new HIV infections among adult population from 2.74 lakh in 2000 to 1.16 lakh in 2011, reflecting the impact of various interventions and scaled-up prevention strategies under the National AIDS Control

Programme (NACP). The trend of annual AIDS deaths is showing a steady decline since roll out of the free Anti-Retroviral Therapy (ART) programme in India in 2004; it is estimated that around 1.5 lakh lives have been saved due to ART till 2011 (NACO,2008).

The central effect of AIDS is a dramatic depletion of a specific subset of T lymphocytes known as the CD4 T cells. AIDS, however, is not simply a virus affecting the immune system. It may also refer to a neuropsychiatric disorder. HIV and AIDS patients develop neurological and psychiatric symptoms which are believed to be due to a direct infection of the brain by HIV. AIDS patients may sometimes demonstrate affective, cognitive, and motor symptoms even before the diagnosis of AIDS is made. HIV disease is a chronic condition in which the asymptomatic phase, i.e., without symptoms, may last form many years. Although most medical interventions are directed towards the control of diseases which occur as a result of the lowered immune function, an increasing range of anti – retroviral drugs which inhibit the replication of HIV and thus tackle the virus directly is now available. Undoubtedly, medical advances in the treatment of HIV disease are being made, and many individuals live longer and survive repeated bouts of illness. However, the length of remission which the new anti- retroviral medications might bring is still unclear. The resulting uncertainty in prognosis increases the emotional burden for those with HIV, even in those who are clinically well and asymptomatyic.

Psychological issues in HIV/AIDS
Many intense, negative psychological reactions have been reported in people with HIV disease (Hedge et al., 1992). The symptoms experienced subsequent to HIV/AIDS diagnosis are given below. It can be seen that anxiety and depression are the most common reaction. Manifestations of anxiety and depression can be categorized as somatic, cognitive, affective   and behavioral as

shown below. People often, but not always experience some symptoms from each category.

Common symptoms associated with Anxiety and Depression

Symptoms	Anxiety	Depression
Somatic (physical)	Increased heart rate fast breathing sweating nausea and diarrhea frequent micturition muscle pains headaches sleep difficulties	Sleep disturbance loss of libido anorexia
Cognitive (thoughts)	Reduced concentration preoccupation with problems catastrophizing	Failure worthlessness unlovable guilt hopelessness
Affective (feelings)	Fear loss of control painc restlessness	Irritability low mood despair lack of energy reduced activity levels

Coming to terms with HIV disease

Even when people suspect the they may be infected with HIV, confirmation of their positivity can come as a shock. Many parallels can be drawn between fatal illnesses, but the former may have to face additional problems, such as the stigma and discrimination attached to gay sexual behaviors, drug use or racial intolerance (King, 1989a). The uncertainty attached to the course of HIV disease, its poor long- term prognosis and the ever- changing recommendations for optimum medication regimes can cause great distress. Many people are concerned that should they develop symptomatic disease they will not be able to cope with its physical symptoms, nor with the frank explanations or elaborate excuses necessary to explain their condition to friends, relatives or employers. So it does not seem surprising that psychological symptoms are frequently seen in those with HIV disease; indeed, it is more remarkable how well so many people cope for so long.

Role of Informational and Mental Health Counseling

Pre- and post- time counseling has two major aims. The first is to prevent further transmission of HIV by helping the individuals maintain sager sex and drug using behaviors. The second is to minimize the distress attached to a positive result. These aims are intricately related, so counseling aims towards supporting an individual may well also benefit society in general. Counseling involves more simply giving information. Although the provision of accurate, up-to – date information about HIV infection is essential, the counseling process enables people to relate relevant information to their own behaviours and circumstances, and so help them to understand their own level of risk make informed decisions of whether to test. This can be achieved by guiding people thought the problem solving process, i.e., fact finding exploring options, decision making, accepting consequences, finding practical assistance and providing further support as necessary. The use of leaflets or videos to provide information may be beneficial, but cannot replace discussion.

Pre- test counseling aims to ensure that individuals are fully informed about the meaning of a positive test result and its implications and are prepared to cope should their result be positive. This information should be given to the patient by an expert who has been involved with the patient right from the beginning of the session. It is important to assess the internal resources and support system available to the patient before informing about the positive findings. It helps the patients to cope better with the disease.

Post- test counseling provides an opportunity for patients who test positive to explore ways in which quality of life can be enhanced while living with HIV infection, and for discussion of the prevention of further spread of infection. The need for confidentiality is of prime importance in testing for HIV, to maintain people's trust, to respect their rights and to prevent discrimination against them.

Goals of pre test counselling

- Explain what the test means and what it does not tell
- Alert to possible ramifications of a positive test result
- Assess personal risk
- Discuss the advantages and disadvantages of knowing HIV status
- Develop coping strategies
- Identify social support, who to tell and why to be circumspect
- Educate in safer sex and safer injecting practices
- Explain confidentiality of test result.

Goals of pre test counseling

- Focus on the reason for the session
- Give clear, simple, unambiguous information
- Clarify the meaning of an HIV positive test
- Expect emotional reactions: shock, denial, anxiety, anger
- Address individual's immediate concerns
- Identify and address issues of immediate importance, e.g., who to and who not to tell; who to use for support; safer sex and injecting practices
- Provide a lifeline, e.g., 24- hour helpline telephone number and written information about HIV, giving details of services available
- Give a further appointment within a few days.

Psychological symptoms have been documented at all stages of infection. Following a positive HIV antibody test, patients commonly voice many fears and often show symptoms of psychological distress. To prepare people for receiving appositive test result and minimize associated distress, it is recommended that pre- and post- test counseling be available for all those considering having an HIV antibody test.

Stress, Coping Skills and Social Support

A number of models have been proposed to explain how psychological and physical dysfunctions are related to induced stress. For example, Lazarus and Folkman (1984) conceptualize coping as constantly changing cognitive and behavioural efforts to manage external and/ or internal demands that are appraised as taxing or exceeding the resources of the person', and that stress occurs when the perceived biological, psychological and social resources available are not sufficient to meet the demands of the situation. It is well documented that stress, or non- coping, is frequently accompanied by various emotional reaction such as fear, anxiety, depression and anger. Lazarus and Flokman's model suggests that the costs and benefits of possible coping behaviors are evaluated, and that the coping behavior perceived a most beneficial is then adopted. There is evidence that an appraisal of the threat presented by a stressor could be 'buffered' by the availability and extent of social support systems (Cohen and Wills, 1985), the individual's perceived control over the situation and the coping style employed. According to this model, the way people deal with HIV disease will depend upon their understanding and interpretation of the event, stresses experienced, the coping options they perceive as available, and on meditating factors such as the perceived availability of social support and the coping strategies they finally adopt.

The role of precipitating factors in relations to stress is well established. Lovett et al., (1993) suggested that life events increase psychological distress in people with HIV disease. Hedge et al., (1992), examining individuals presenting in crisis to an HIV psychology service, found the most frequently reported preceding events to be personal illness (39 per cent), bereavement (30 per cent), fears concerning disclosure of HIV status (23 per cent), issues surrounding testing (17 per cent), dilemmas concerning medication (17 per cent) and child difficulties (10 per cent). Eighty0 nine per cent of crises were preceded by two or more major events or dilemmas. These data safest that it is the cumulative stress level which leads to an inability to copy, and emphasize the need to recognize the impact of multiple, concurrent problems even if not are directly related to HIV.

There is also evidence (Hedge et al., 1993) that strategies used to cope with HIV disease affect the psychological distress levels experienced. Adaptive coping styles included active coping strategies, such as the seeking of emotional support and problem focused coping and the maintenance of a high level of self- esteem. Increased denial, emotional and behavioral disengagement, hopelessness and less positive reframing experiences were associated with increased psychological morbidity.

Psychological Intervention Strategies
Given the high levels of psychological distress experienced by individual with HIV disease, it is imperative to consider ways of minimizing the effects of stressors. This section will explore a cognitive- behavioral model, describe some intervention studies and consider some common issue and dilemmas which can lead to distress.

Cognitive – Behavioral Model
There is a substantial body of evidence which suggests that therapy based on Beck's cognitive- behavioral model of treatment can benefit those with psychological symptomatology. This model rests on three assumptions.

- Thought determine emotions and behavior
- Unrealistic and negative thoughts lead to emotional disorder
- Decreasing unrealistic and negative thoughts and increasing realistic positive thoughts reduce emotional symptomatology.

A common misapprehension is that cognitive behavior therapy is the encouragement of positive thinking. In fact it comprises a number of techniques which address dysfunctional cognitions and behaviors within a structured therapy session. For example, because many realities for those with HIV infection are negative, the technique of decat-astrophization' is used. This is a process which attempts to separate the reality from the accompanying global negative feelings, and allows the person to explore coping alternatives, thought positive reframing. A thought such as 'I'll never be well enough to return to work' may be realistic when expressed by an individual with HIV disease. If the corollary is 'so I'll never be happy again', then though depressive could result, whereas the follow- up thought' so I'll have plenty of time for reading' can be part of a positive, coping strategy. Thus, decatastrophization and positive reframing can play a major role in preventing a server depressive or anxiety response.

List of Cognitive – Behavioral Intervention
- Relaxation training and breathing exercises
- Activity scheduling
- Thought stopping
- Reality resting
- Decatastrophization
- Positive reframing
- Problem solving
- Development of long- term and intermediate goals

The problem solving approach aims to support individuals in making informed decisions about their present difficulties and to equip them with the general skills and strategies necessary for dealing with future problems.

Intervention Studies on CBT

George (1988) examined patients with HIV disease 6-12 months after individual, cognitive- behavioral interventions. She found a significant reduction in distress and sustained improvements in anxiety, and depression. Similarly, Hedge et al., (1993) reported increases in self- esteem and decreases in anxiety and depression following an intervention aimed at increasing coping skills. A number of group interventions have been successful in reducing stress, improving coping skills and improving quality of life (Lamping et al., 1993; Kelly et al., 1993). Hedge and Glover (1990) showed that educational groups not only provided information, but also relieved distress and enhanced mutual support.

Coping with Grief

There is no 'correct' way to grieve, nor any set time after which the grieving should have ceased. Models of the normal grieving process (Kubler-Ross, 1970; Worden, 1992) have been built from descriptions of common reactions to death and the tasks, stages or phases which individuals typically encounter while learning to live with the realities of death. However, the reaction of an individual to a particular death will be affected by the circumstances in which it occurs. Consideration of the models suggests that some ways of coping with death may be more beneficial than others.

Bereavement in the context of HIV presents some unique features. For example, those who die are usually young and the highest rate of mortality is in the age range of 20- 40 years. Furthermore, death is often the last of many losses, as HIV infection may have already brought the loss of relationships, sex, employment, control, a future, hope and health. In addition, those bereaved by HIV frequently are themselves HIV-positive. If bereavement or its psychological sequelae has an adverse effect on the immune system, then it could prove hazardous to health. Folkman *et al.* (1994) have described the patterns of distress experienced by caregivers during illness and death. They found that prior to the death of a partner, HIV positive caregivers were less distressed than those not infected, while after the death the infected partners showed more distress. A possible explanation is that those who are HIV positive view the experience as a model of their own death. First, they empathize with the patient; afterwards they realize they may face a similar experience alone, as their own infection makes it.less likely that they will find a new partner, Lennon, Martin and Dean (1990) report the intensity of grief during bereavement to be related to the involvement in caretaking during end-stage disease, and to the adequacy of practical and emotional support given to the caregiver during this time.

Most people experiencing grief will not need professional help; the support of friends and relatives and general guidance from the social or health care providers who have given support to the recently deceased will be adequate. Reassurance that it is natural to grieve, together with an explanation that this may involve exploring positive and negative feelings about the deceased, dealing with emotions such as anger, guilt and hopelessness and anticipation of the problems and necessary changes which the death may bring about, can be useful- For people bereaved through HIV, peer support groups for partners, friends and relatives, organized by volunteers and community groups, complement services provided by health professionals and social workers.

When the stigma attached to HIV leads people to fear rejection and so hide their losses, isolate themselves and not make use of available social support, there is an increased chance of abnormal grief response. Abnormal grieving is usually categorized by grief reactions of abnormal intensity which persist over time with little evidence of change. Guided mourning (Mawson, Marks and Ramn, 1981), increasing adaptive coping skills and increasing appropriate social support can assist the grief process. Occasionally, a death will precipitate a frank psychiatric response. Appropriate psychiatric intervention, e.g. for a depressed or psychotic stare, as well as grief management will then be necessary.

Another facet of AIDS-related bereavement, the social loss, was described by Dean *et al.* (1988), who reported multiple bereavement in a large cohort ot gay men in San Francisco. Ninety-five per cent of the sample reported HIV~related loss, with an average of 6.2 HIV-relatcd deaths each. With increasing numbers of AIDS related deaths, McKusick (1991) reported increasing distress involving:

- Psychological and emotional numbness
- Shrinking away from friends and resources
- Symptoms of complicated bereavement (inordinate guilt, calcified anger, rage, indifference)
- depression.

He described a cycle of negative impact: deaths led to a decrease in the available social support which resulted in higher levels of depression in those with HIV disease, which had the effect of less self-care which increased the likelihood of mortality, etc. To combat the effects of multiple bereavement, the adoption of a community-wide coping programme to enable people to stay involved rather than distance themselves from the problem, and to find some form of social support which promotes discharge of anxieties and renewal of vigour. The use of public ritual, e.g. annual candlelight ceremonies to mourn the people lost to HIV, can support communities in reaffirming their capability to overcome these feelings of loss and to remain empowered.

Burnout

The term 'burnout' is used to characterize a syndrome which can develop when stresses are not recognized and addressed (Maslach, 1982). Maslach and Jackson (1981) defined burnout as a combination of emotional exhaustion, depersonalization and a reduced sense of personal accomplishment.

Factors which have been identified as increasing the levels of stress staff experienced while working with people with HIV disease are as follows

- Younger age of the patient
- Stress level of the patient
- Number of his/her dependents
- Younger age of the staff
- Identification with the patient
- Involvement of the patient
- External coping resources of the staff
- Lack of internal coping resources like knowledge and skills of the staff
- Organizational stressors
- Stigma of working with HIV/AIDS patients and
- Disagreement over patient treatment

The question of whether AIDS presents unique burdens to health care staff is not easily answered. Many of the factors contributing to stress are experienced by care workers in other fields such as oncology and cystic fibrosis. The greater patient dependency in HIV units necessitated the need for greater contact between the nurse and patient, and increased the emotional intensity of the work. Bennett et al (1992) investigated factors which could be associated with burnout. They found grief not to be predictive of burnout, but that greater work-related grief was experienced when carers identified closely with patients. Burnout was associated with an absence of internal coping strategies, and with a reliance on external coping strategies, e.g. excessive alcohol or drug usage. Older, more experienced carers were less likely to experience burnout.

Strategies to Minimize Burnout

To minimize burnout, strategies are needed to focus on both the individual's coping skills and on the organization's attempt to minimize stressors. In line with the findings that intensity of work rather than overall length of time working on an HIV unit contributed to stress levels (Bennett, Michie& Kippax. 1991), time our techniques (e.g. rotating with staff in the genito-urinary medicine clinic) could be adopted. To utilize the coping strategies of those who are older and who have more experience, increasing the opportunities for informal sharing of problem might be beneficial. Alternatively, the provision of staff support groups could facilitate exchange of information and coping strategies between experienced and inexperienced staff".

When patients are seen for a long time by a relatively small group of care staff, close emotional involvement with patients frequently occurs. Specific training in strategics aimed at expressing warmth and empathy while maintaining professional boundaries has been suggested to reduce emotional stress (Bennett *et al.,* 199 1).

To facilitate carers in the above, organizational change may be required. This may include

- Assessment of job requirements and available resources
- Task planning
- Staff development, education and training
- Enhancing communication systems
- Provision of formal support
- Enhancing informal communications and appreciation
- Reviewing job structure and workload.

NEUROPSYCHOLOGICAL COMPLICATION OF DISEASE

The neuropsychological effects of HIV disease are many and varied (Grant, 1990), and can result from either the direct effect of HIV on the central nervous system of from secondary complications of immune deficiency (e.g. cerebral opportunistic infections such as toxoplasmosis, progressive multi- focal leuconencephalopathy and lymphoma).

Cognitive impairment has been reported in people with asymptomatic HIV but this is unusual. Most cases being seen in advanced disease states (McArthur et al., 1993). The pattern of cognitive deficits which emerges in late stage disease shows impairment consistent with some features of sub cortical dementia, including memory impairment and decline in fine motor speed, concentration, problem solving and visuo- special ability (Navia 1990). The incidence of HIV associated dementia is reported to be around 7 per cent (Janssen et al, 1990) and the prevalence cited as ranging from 2.6-16 per cent (Meadows et al., 1993a).

Family Interventions

In most instances, an individual's AIDS diagnosis affects family members. This group may include a spouse or partner, children, extended family, support network and family of origin. Family systems risk fractures as they attempt to manage the enormous impact of AIDS on their lives. Lack of social and financial support risk the family disruption. The overall goal of family intervention includes enhancing the ability of the family to support each other, to focus on immediate crises, to assist grieving process, to encourage resolution of long standing conflicts and to decrease each member's isolation by facilitation socil support outside the family system. Psychotherapists utilize individual therapy, couple therapy family therapy, home visits and group interventions to address these goals.

SPIRITUALITY AND HIV/AIDS

Facing the mystery and suffering of HIV illness, both patient and therapist may turn to religion, spirituality and concepts of God in their efforts to find solace, understanding and emotional healing. Often, the issues of connection to a greater reality, blame, shame or guilt based on religious beliefs and the role of God become prominent issues in psychotherapy. The patient may long for connections with higher powers like God and try to search for new senses of meaning. These efforts can provide a sense of belonging and connection to a larger reality. And can create new emotional hurts or remind clients of old strictures and messages of guilt and punishment. It is important to explore the patient's religious life in the context of pre HIV life and culture to understand his/her religious feelings in the context of HIV. Spirituality can help the patient to foster forgiveness and healing if there is a strong guilt in the patient. Spirituality can help the patient to develop hope in them and finding new meaning in experiences becomes pro active and altering one's attitude and cognitions. Maintaining hope requires reframing and redefining. The hope needs to be associated with day to day accomplishments, mastery skills and events to enhance feelings of being hopeful.

DETOXIFYING DEATH AND DYING

Thoughts of death and dying evoke primitive and intense feelings in everyone. Most people, however, use a "functional denial" to put these emotions aside so that they can continue to live their lives. Despite their constant presence, patients invariably try to avoid these topics, because they are so painful and frightening. Well-meaning (but equally terrified) family and friends usually collude with this avoidance due to their own anxiety about losing a loved one. Consequently, patients are left alone with their worst fears and fantasies. In the absence of a place where the patient can reveal and contemplate these terrifying images, they will inevitably experience negative emotions that will compromise their emotional well-being. Patients who are left to ruminate about their death are unable to fully participate in life or enjoy much of living. Addressing death and related issues in a direct manner has the effect of decreasing the fear and anxiety that normally go along with it. Through addressing these fears and anxieties, patients learn that they can both tolerate such thoughts and that there may be things they can do for themselves to moderate their anxiety. Patients frequently find it an immense relief to simply be able to talk about death and dying in an unrestrained, explicit way. Helping patients break this particular subject down into smaller, more manageable parts diminishes the fear and anxiety associated with it.

HIV/AIDS AND BEHAVIOR CONTROL AS PREVENTION STRATEGY

Prevention of infection with the AIDS (Acquired Immunodeficiency Syndrome) virus requires people to exercise influence over their own motivation and behavior. Social efforts designed to control the spread of AIDS have centred mainly on informing the public on how the human immunodeficiency virus (HIV) is transmitted and how to safeguard against such infection. It is widely assumed that if people are informed adequately about the AIDS threat they will take appropriate self-protective action. Heightened awareness and knowledge of health risks are important preconditions for self-directed change. To achieve self-directed change, people need to be given not only reasons to alter risky habits but also the means and resources to do so. Effective self-regulation of behavior is not achieved by an act of will. It requires certain skills in self-motivation and self-guidance (Bandura, 1986). Moreover, there is a difference between possessing coping skills and being able to use them effectively and consistently under difficult circumstances. Success, therefore, requires not only skills, but also strong self-belief in one's capabilities to exercise personal control.

Numerous studies have been conducted linking perceived self-efficacy to health-promoting and health impairing behavior (Bandura, 1986, 1989; O'Leary,1985). The results show that perceived efficacy can affect every phase of personal change-whether people even consider changing their health habits, how hard they try should they choose to do so, how much they change, and how well they maintain the changes they have achieved. In addition to influencing health habits, perceived coping inefficacy increases vulnerability to stress and depression and activates biochemical changes that can affect various facets of immune function.

In managing sexuality, people have to exercise influence over themselves as well as over others. This requires self-regulatory skills in guiding and motivating one's actions. Self-regulation operates through internal standards, affective reactions to one's conduct, use of motivating self incentives, and other forms of cognitive self-guidance. Self-regulatory skills thus form an integral part of risk-reduction capabilities. They partly determine the social situations into which people get themselves, how well they navigate through them, and how effectively they can resist social inducements to potentially risky behavior. It is easier to wield control over preliminary choice behavior that may lead to troublesome social situations than to try to extricate oneself from such situations. This is because the antecedent phase involves mainly anticipatory motivators which are amenable to cognitive control; the entanglement phase includes stronger social inducements to engage in high-risk behavior which are less easily manageable.

The ability to learn by social modeling provides a highly effective method for increasing human knowledge and skills. A special power of modeling is that it can transmit simultaneously knowledge and valuable skills to large numbers of people through the medium of videotape modeling. Knowledge of modeling processes identifies a number of factors that can be used to enhance the instructive power of modeling. Applications of modeling principles to AIDS prevention would focus on how to manage interpersonal situations and one's own behavior in ways that afford protection against infection with the AIDS virus. Both self-regulatory and risk-reduction strategies for dealing with a variety of situations would be modeled to convey general guides that can be applied and adjusted to fit changing circumstances.

CONCLUSION

The emotional reactions to infection with HIV have been well documented. HIV is associated with multiple stressors including physical illness, bereavement, psychological issues like depression, anger, anxiety etc and medication dilemmas. An individual's ability to cope is associated with the cumulative stress experienced and the perceived available social support. Further work on the interaction between stressors and the functioning of the immune system is needed. There is evidence that psychological strategies which develop coping skills and which enable people to mobilize social support are beneficial in the short term. In relation to this, it is important to recognize the effect which bereavement from HIV related deaths is having on communities, traditionally those who have provided social support. It becomes essential to address the coping skills of the care givers and providing psychological interventions to HIV/AIDS patients along with medical interventions for better recovery and improving quality of life of these patients.

REFERENCES

Dilley,J.W.,Pies, C.,& Helquist,M. (1989). *Face to Face: A guide to AIDS Counseling.* AIDS Health Project Publication, San Francisco, CA

Hedge,B.,Patrak, J., Sherr,L.,Sichel,T., Glover,L.,&Slaughter,J.(1992). 'Psychological crises in HIV infection' *VIII International AIDS Conference*, Amsterdam.

King, M.B.(1989a). Psychological status of 192 out patients and HIV infections and AIDS. *British Journal of Psychiatry, 154,* 237-242

National AIDS Control Organization. (2008). Report by the Indian government's AIDS organization. Retrieved from http// www.avert.org/india-hiv-aids-statistics on Feb 2nd, 2011.

National AIDS Control Organization: Annual Report (2013-2014). Department of AIDS Control, Ministry of Health and Family Welfare, Government of India

Rabkin, J., Remien,R., Katoff,L., & Williams, J. (1993). Suicidality in AIDS long term survivors: What is the evidence? *AIDS Care,5,* 410-411

Winiarski, M.G.(1991). *AIDS-Related Psychotherapy,* Pergamon Press: New York

Knowledge and Attitude Regarding HIV/AIDS among College Students of Kulgam Jammu and Kashmir

Dr. Abdul Bari Naik[26]*, Abdul Raffie Naik[27], Tanveer Ahmad Lone[28]

ABSTRACT

The current study was an effort to know the knowledge and attitude regarding HIV/AIDS among college students of Kulgam Dist., Jammu and Kashmir. Inadequate knowledge and negative attitudes are major hindrances to prevent the spread of HIV. Studying the HIV-related knowledge and attitudes is a promising area of inquiry

The age of college students is a critical age in which the probability of becoming the victim of HIV/AIDS is more imminent. Therefore, the purpose of the study is to assess HIV/AIDS related knowledge and understand how much percentage of said population are having knowledge about this disease so that further interventions can be planned. The study was conducted on 515 college student of govt. degree college Kulgam. The data was collected through self-administered questionnaire. The questionnaire was composed of AIDS related knowledge, aptitude and behaviour question items. The results of the study showed that students had adequate knowledge of the basic facts about AIDS, the transmission of HIV and how they can protect themselves was found to co-exist with some misconceptions.

Keywords: HIV-AIDS, Knowledge and aptitude.

[26] Assistant Professor Govt. Degree College Kulgam
[27] MS.C Clinical and Counselling Psychology CUK
[28] M.Phil. Women's Education MANUU Hyderabad.
*Corresponding Author

"HIV/AIDS" is the abbreviation of *"human immune Deficiency Virus/Acquired Immune-Deficiency Syndrome"*. AIDS is a fatal disease described variously as modern plague, scourge, distressing disease, and insidious biological disaster. It has emerged as an unprecedented pandemic cutting across all boundaries - International, Socioeconomic, Sex, Age, and Race. AIDS is already well-known in several countries of the world. Its exponential progression and tremendous impact on mankind is still frightening. HIV (Human Immune Deficiency Virus) catches persons usually in their prime youth. Adolescents and youth need information in order to make such responsible choices in terms of sexual behaviour/relationship. They also need to integrate and personalize this information or knowledge so that they can make healthy choices. Young people learn a great deal from each other and by sharing ideas and experiences amongst themselves. Peer influence is a great motivating factor in the adoption of specific behaviour patterns. Therefore, correct information and values imparted to one group of young people will be passed on to the other young people. Young people who have developed greater self-esteem and mutually supportive relationships are less vulnerable to peer and other pressures.

AIDS is a world health problem of extraordinary scale and extreme urgency. It emerged as one of the most important public health issues of the late twentieth and early twenty- first centuries and is now one of the leading causes of global morbidity and mortality. For prevention from such disease one needs to have an adequate knowledge, few reasons for HIV/AIDS education are

I. To prevent new infections from taking place

Prevention of infection can be described as a two-pronged approach: Firstly giving people information about HIV/AIDS transmission modes and how people can protect themselves from infection.

Secondly, people must be taught how to use this information to use and act on it practically – how to get and use condoms, how to suggest and practice safer sex, how to prevent infection via accidental exposure or when injecting drugs.

II.   To improve quality of life for HIV positive people

AIDS education is often seen as being something that should be targeted only at people who are HIV negative in order to prevent them from becoming infected. When AIDS education with HIV positive people is considered at all it is frequently seen only in terms of preventing new infections by teaching HIV positive people about the importance of not passing on the virus.

An important and commonly neglected aspect of AIDS education with HIV positive people is enabling and empowering them to improve their quality of life by advocating healthy lifestyle adjustments. HIV positive people have varying educational needs, but among them are the need to be able to access medical services, access to anti-retroviral drugs and the need to be able to find appropriate emotional and practical counseling, support and help.

III.   To reduce stigma and discrimination

There exist a great deal of fear and stigmatization of people who are HIV positive. Ignorance, resentment and ultimately, anger often accompany this fear. Sometimes the results of prejudice and fear can be extreme, with HIV positive people being burnt to death in India, and many families being forced to flee their homes around the globe when neighbors discover a family member's positive status.

Discrimination against HIV positive people can help the epidemic to spread, because people are fearful of being tested for HIV, and then they are more likely to pass the infection to someone else without knowing.

"Peer education gives people the opportunity to ask questions outside an academic environment and with someone who isn't an authority figure"

METHODOLOGY

Methodology of the study

This study is undertaken to make an attempt for understanding and knowing about the knowledge and attitude of college students of Govt. degree college kulgam regarding HIV/AIDS.

Objectives:

The study will be conducted with the following objectives:

1. To measure the level of knowledge of students of Govt. degree college Kulgam regarding HIV/AIDS.
2. To assess the attitude of students of Govt. degree college Kulgam regarding HIV/AIDS.
3. To measure the level of knowledge about modes of transmission of HIV/ADIS.

Population:

The population for the present study consists of students studying in Govt. degree college Kulgam pursuing Graduation. The age range of the population is 16 – 25 years, studying inKulgam dist.

Sources of the data:

For the study, only primary data was used. The data required for the study was collected using questionnaires that were distributed among the sample chosen from the population that were the students studying in Govt. Degree College Kulgam.

Procedure:

The questionnaire was administered under classroom conditions to students without the presence of their teachers. The participants were welcomed and rapport was established. The researcher gave brief information about the purpose of the study and informed consent had been taken from the participants. Respondents were asked to complete an anonymous questionnaire about various aspects about knowledge and attitude regarding HIV/AIDS. They were also told that the questionnaire would be kept strictly confidential and anonymous. It was emphasized that the exercise was wholly voluntary and that individuals were free to discontinue the questionnaire at any point. After the questionnaire were completed, participants were debriefed and a short group AIDS prevention counselling was offered.

RESULTS AND DISCUSSION

Table: 1 Frequency distribution of study participant's age group

Age group	Frequency	Percentage
17-19	233	45.2
20-22	189	36.6
23-25	93	18

Table 1 shows the distribution of age group of the participants in the present study. The total number of participants were 515 under which there are 233 (45.2%) under age group 17-19, 189(36.6%) under 20-22 age group and 93(18%) under 23-25 age group.

Table 2 Awareness among participants on HIV/AIDS

Total population under study:	515
Percentage who had heard about HIV/AIDS	96.69%
Perceptions about the causative agent/factor	
Germ/Virus:	63.10%
Insects/bad air/stale food:	25.43%
No idea at all:	11.47%
Knowledge about established modes of transmission	
a) Correct awareness	
Use of infected syringes	82.3%

Sexual contact	84%
Use of infected blood	69.30%
Sharing of toothbrushes/blades	53.8%
Mother to child	28%
b) False perceptions about spread of HIV/AIDS	
Handshake	9%
Eating with the patient	24%
Use of fomites	15%
Source of awareness	
Electronic media	36.13%
Print material (including textbooks)	28.60%
Friends	19%
Teachers	12%
Parents	1.97%
Siblings	2.33%

Among the participants only 3.31% of population are those who do not know about the term HIV/AIDS. 11.47% do not have any idea about the causative agent/factor.9% of participants have false perception that HIV/AIDS can spread by handshake.24% about eating with the patient and 15%'s perception believe that use of fomites spread disease. Source of awareness about the disease is mostly from electronic media and printing material.

Table 3: Attitude towards the HIV/AIDS and its Victims

Ever discussed HIV/AIDS with	
Friends	41.70%
Sister	8.80%
Teachers	15.30%
Brothers	1.5%
Father	0.80%
Mother	0.22%
Population that should be targeted for HIV/AIDSeducation:	

Incorrect / no knowledge	23%
Correct perceptions	68%
Parents of adolescents	3.70%
Adolescents (Boys and girls)	18.7%
All adults	6%
Attitude towards patients of HIV/AIDS	
Hospitalization and isolate	48%
Treat as outpatient with extra precautions	34%
Ostracize/ shun/ abandon/isolate	
boycott/expel from school	3.3%
Give necessary support	5%
No opinion	12%

Table no: 3 shows that most of the participants have discussed about the disease with friends and a little number had discussed with their teachers. Very few participants had discussed about the disease with their parents.

Population that should be targeted for HIV/AIDS education according this study is 23% who do not have any information about HIV/ADIS or have incorrect knowledge. The attitude of the population towards the patients of HIV/AIDS is a big concern which is due to the less knowledge about the concept of the disease.

The studied population comprised of 17-25 year old college students from Govt degree college Kulgam. The results, however, revealed a good awareness among the respondents. The main source of AIDS-awareness for adolescents was the media, especially the T.V., followed by print media (including textbooks). This is suggestive of the fact that incorporation of HIV/AIDS as part of the curriculum has not made the desired impact. There may be two possible reasons for this; one, the teachers' reluctance to discuss the subject with the students and second being the education system itself which allows such a crucial subject like HIV/AIDS to get bypassed from the curriculum. In our study, teachers were cited as an important source of awareness by a mere 15 percent of the respondents.

Friends, who because of their own ignorance and misconceptions could be dangerously misguiding, formed the 3rd most important source of information. Discussions around HIV/AIDS were most frequently made with friends followed by siblings. Very ironically, a mere 0.22 percent could discuss HIV with their mothers which reflected the prevalent parochial parental attitudes. Matters pertaining to sex, sexuality and reproduction continue to be a taboo in conservative societies. The present findings are supported by data from NFHS-2 and those generated by ICMR-interventional programmes for adolescents which reported that only 15 percent of the mothers conversed with their daughters on the subject of menstrual cycle; 66-73 percent felt shy to talk on the subject indicating the extent of inhibitions we share in communicating with our young adolescents.

CONCLUSION

The present study shows a dismal picture of HIV awareness and attitude among the educated population. The study highlighted some misconceptions about HIV transmission, knowledge intolerant attitudes, stigma and discrimination towards PLHIV, which need to be addressed. HIV/AIDS-related education programmes should include specific interventions to change practices, along with knowledge and attitudes. Future research involving nationally representative samples for male and female, college-attending and out-of-college adolescents could contribute substantially to HIV/AIDS prevention.

The results also indicate that carefully planned information, education and communication can be used to correct misunderstandings about HIV/AIDS and its prevention practices. Mass media or public media campaigns can raise the bar of knowledge in students. AIDS awareness in curriculum should be included at all levels of education as researchers supported the idea of school-based education of HIV/AIDS. These curricula are instrumental in increasing students' knowledge about AIDS, dispelling misconceptions about casual contact as a route of disease transmission; and decreasing student's fear and vulnerability about having classmates with AIDS or HIV infection especially at college level. Similarly, education has been recommended as the best line of defence against the spread of the AIDS.

REFERENCES

Bandawe, C.R. & Foster, D. (1996). AIDS-related beliefs, attitudes and intentions among
    Malawian students in three secondary schools. AIDS Care, 8(2), 223-232

Iqbal, M. (2015). HIV/AIDS and Social Exclusion in Kashmir. hyderabad, Telangana, india.

IIPS/ORC Marco: National Family Health Survey of India 1998-99(2002). NFHS-2;
    J& K, October, p. 149-55

Kapiga, S.H., Nachtigal, G. & Hunter, D.J. (1991). Knowledge of Aids among secondary
    Schoolpupils in Bugamoyo and Dar-Es-Salaam, Tanzania. AIDS, 5(3), 325-328.

Puja, G.K. & Kassimoto, T. (1994). Girls in education ad pregnancy at school. In Z.T.
    Masabo & R. Liljestrom (Eds), Chelewa, chelewa: The dilemma of teenage girls
    (pp. 54-75). Stockholm: Scandivavian Institute of African

Stout, J.W. & Rivara, F.P. (1989). Schools and sex education: Does it work? Paediatrics,
    83, 375-379.

Wilson, D., Greenspan, R. & Wilson, C. (1989). Knowledge about AIDS and
    Self-reported behaviour among Zimbabwean secondary school pupils. Social Science and Medicne, 28(9), 957-961.

Emergence and Social Stigmatization of HIV/AIDS in Kashmir Valley

Abdul Basit Naik[29]*, Abdul Bari Naik[29]

ABSTRACT

The study was done to enlighten on the emergence and social stigmatization of HIV/AIDS in Kashmir valley. The simple size of the study was taken as 50 through the purposive random sampling. The aim of the study was to know the mode of transmission of HIV infection. Since the HIV prevalence is considerable low in Kashmir as compared to other states of India and the factors responsible for such low prevalence to HIV/AIDS are not known, but definitely this is being attributed to strong socio-religious factors prevalent in Kashmir society. The primary goal of this study is to find out the emergence of HIV/AIDS in Kashmir, gender difference, material status, age, locality, social stigma and discrimination experienced by these respondents in Kashmir valley. Majority of HIV positive patients belonged to males. Results also show that HIV infected persons in Kashmir valley are non-locals. Transmission of infection was through sexual contact in 80 % followed by homosexual transmission in 2 %. Vertical transmission and blood transfusion accounted in 2% cases each. One of the reason may be happen due to lack of proper knowledge about the disease. So Government departments and institutions, Non-Government Organizations and counseling centers should spread awareness about the disease with rejuvenated zeal.

Keywords: HIV-AIDS, Kashmir, Emergence

AIDS is an acronym of *"acquired immune deficiency syndrome"* which is a fatal disease described variously as modern plague, modern scourge, devastating disease, insidious microbiological

---

[29] Research Scholar, Maulana Azad National Urdu University, Gochibowli, Hyderabad
*Corresponding Author

bomb. It has emerged as an unprecedented pandemic cutting across all boundaries international, socio-economic, age, race and gender. AIDS emerged as one of the most important public health issues of late twentieth and early twenty first centuries and is now one of the leading causes of global morbidity and mortality (Wallace, 2014). AIDS is also considered a socio-cultural issue because when this epidemic emerged in 1981, it was perceived as a deadly disease that was transmissible from person to person, as well as closely associated with historically disenfranchised groups and culturally and historically taboos and issues such as sexual orientation, drug use, unethical sex, prostitution, commercial sex workers etc.

The combination of these factors led to societal hostility from community and other immediate social groups as well as slow response by state, federal, and country governments. Although both knowledge of HIV/AIDS and government response has increased across the time in almost all societies now, but the stigma and hostility still persists more than 30 years later (Tomaszewski, 2012).

Srinagar is the largest city of the J&K state (Jammu and Kashmir) with population crossing over one million has been placed in low prevalence state, but still it is at a high risk due to presence of more than five lakh security personnel, tourists, religious pilgrimages and migrant population coming for work from other parts of the country. The specific objective of this study is to find out clinical profile as well as the demographic and epidemiological characteristics of attendees whose samples were seropositive for HIV/Aids.

The history of HIV/AIDS is short one, and the origins of HIV are disputed yet since it was first reported just over thirty years ago, it has became one of the leading cause of death throughout the world. In 1986, the first known case of HIV was diagnosed by Dr. Suniti Solmon amongst female sex workers in Chennai. At that time foreigners in India were travelling in and out of the country. It is thought that these foreigners were the ones responsible for the first infections in the country. Although the prevalence of HIV in Kashmir is very less as compared to most of the Indian states, the first case of HIV in Kashmir was identified in the same year (1986) as in India. It was a German returned business man who had got the virus somewhere outside India and died in the same year. Since then there have been many cases; some unidentified and asymptomatic, but the total registrations have not even crossed 230 as yet.

Jammu and Kashmir state AIDS Prevention and Control Society (JKSACS) implements National AIDS control program since 1999 as per National pattern mainly with the help of health and medical education department, and other Govt. departments, Non-Government organizations, community based organizations and civil society for controlling and preventing the spread of HIV/AIDS in the state.

AIDS Prevention and Control Society (ACS), Jammu and Kashmir has 3492 people living with HIV. Jammu division has highest number of HIV positive with 90% of these cases, while Kashmir with only 13% of HIV positive cases detected so far. This puts the total number of HIV positive cases in Kashmir division at 452 in 2011-12 (International AIDS Society, 2010: 45).

Jammu and Kashmir and HIV/AIDS

J&K has unique geographical and socio-economic characteristics that have made the state vulnerable in respect to the spread of HIV/AIDS. Some of the important factors which are contributing to spread of HIV/AIDS are:

1. J&K being a tourist place, visitors from all over the world visit J&K especially Kashmir valley.
2. High concentration of Indian security forces, they keep getting transferred from one state to another state like Karnataka, Maharashtra, Tamil Nadu and other southern

states to Jammu and Kashmir , can bring the HIV infection from those high prevalence states.

3. Migrant laborers who come from different states such as U.P Bihar, Nepal, west Bengal etc to Kashmir, bring HIV.
4. Long distance truck drivers and their helpers are considered as a vulnerable bridge for HIV transmission in the Kashmir valley.

METHODOLOGY:

Aim. The current study tries to highlight the emergence and stigma related to HIV/AIDS patients and the main causal factors which are responsible for spreading HIV/AIDS in the Kashmir valley.

Objectives:

The study has been done on the objectives mentioned below:

1. To study the historical background and emergence of HIV/AIDS in Kashmir valley.

2. To study the main variables responsible for HIV/AIDS in the Kashmir valley.

3. To study the distribution of people living with HIV/AIDS in terms of gender.

4. To study the distribution of people living with HIV/AIDS in terms of local and non local.

5. To study the distribution of people living with HIV/AIDS in terms of age.

6. To study the distribution of people living with HIV/AIDS in terms of marital status.

7. To study the mode of HIV/AIDS transmission (local Kashmir).

Universe of study:

For the current study Kashmir valley has been chosen as study area. Kashmir is the summer capital of Jammu and Kashmir State which consists of 10 districts namely Anantnag, Baramulla, Badgam, Bandipora, Kulgam, Kupwara, Pulwama, Shopian, Ganderbal and

Srinagar. Kashmir division had population of 53, 50, 811 as per the census report 2011.The religious composition was 97.16% of Muslims and 2.84% Hindus, Sikhs, Buddhists and others.

Sample of the Study:

Kashmir division has a very less number of HIV/AIDS patients which is around 230 only including those who expired, but the numbers of patients who came to visit ART(Antiretroviral therapy) cell Srinagar on regular basis are around 90 local Kashmiris excluding non Kashmiris. So the sample size was itself described and sought out. Due to some communication gaps a sample size has been minimized to 50 HIV positive persons from both the rural and urban areas of Kashmir were selected randomly for the study.

For the present study the researchers used exploratory research design to draw the relevant inferences. In addition to it Purposive Random Sampling Technique was employed to gather the data from primary respondents. Though the universe for this study was whole Kashmir division but the study was conducted in an ART centre in Sheri Kashmir Institute of Medical Sciences Srinagar (Kashmir) during the year 2014.A semi-structured pre-tested interview schedule was administrated to the these respondents to gather the information, knowledge about means of transmission of the infection, modes of prevention, attitudes towards them from general community for being HIV positive and social stigma.

Data collection:

The data for the current study was carried out by employing the interview schedule and observation as methodological tools. Further, the primary data was supplemented with the secondary data compiled from the books, articles, HIV/AIDS related pamphlets, etc.

The collected information from the field as well as the secondary source has been put into the subject matter in the form of data tables, graphs ,charts, numbers and words .Data has been assessed, analyzed ,tabulated graphed and interpreted systematically with relevant methodology.

RESULTS AND DISCUSSIONS:

Table No. 1: Shows distribution of people living with HIV/AIDS in terms of gender.

Gender	No. of participants	Percentage
Male	31	62
Female	18	36
Transgender	1	2
Total	50	100

Source: ART Centre SKIMS Soura Srinagar June 2014

The above table shows the maximum number of male infections which is about 62 percent and only 18 percent female infections with a negligible 1percent of transgender.

Table No. 2: Shows the distribution of people living with HIV/AIDS in terms of local and non local.

Residence	No. of participants	Percentage
Local	19	38
Non-local	31	62
Total	50	100

Source: ART Centre SKIMS Soura Srinagar June 2014

The above table shows the maximum number of Non-local are infected which is about 62 percent while as locals account for 38percent.

Table No. 3: Shows the distribution of people living with HIV/AIDS in terms of age

Age group (in years)	No. of participants	Percentage
1-10	1	2
11-20	6	12
21-30	20	40
31-40	4	8
41-50	7	14
51-60	11	22
61-70	1	2
Total	50	100

Source: ART Centre SKIMS Soura Srinagar June 2014

The above table shows that the maximum numbers of people having HIV/AIDS are in between 21-30 years of age group i.e. 40 percent and minimum numbers of people having HIV/AIDS are in 1-10 years and 61-70 years of age groups i.e. 2 percent.

Table No.4: Shows the distribution of people living with HIV/AIDS in terms of marital status

Marital status	No. of participants	Percentage
Married	33	66
Unmarried	10	20
Widow/Widower	7	14
Total	50	100

Source: ART Centre SKIMS Soura Srinagar June 2014

The above table shows that the maximum numbers of people having HIV/AIDS are married while as minimum number of people falls in widow/widower category.

Table No.5: Mode of transmission of HIV among people living with HIV/AIDS distribution

Acronyms	Mode of Transmission	Percentage
HS	Heterosexuals	80
MSM	Male sex Male	1
MTC	Mother to child	2
IDU	Intravenous drug users	3
US	Unprotected sex	5
BT	Blood transfusion	2
UK	Unknown	7

Source: ART Centre SKIMS Soura Srinagar June 2014

The above table shows that 80 percent people having HIV/AIDS are heterosexuals while as 5 percent people agree that they have sex without any protection especially condoms and 3 percent people suffers it by intravenous drug and only 2 percent have it through blood transfusion and mother to child by breast feeding. Only 1 percent agrees that it is due to same sex (male to male sex).

The following points are responsible for spreading the HIV/AIDS in Kashmir valley:

1. Kashmir being a tourist place attracts millions of tourists from different parts of world which may be one of the main reasons for transmitting HIV/AIDS in the valley.
2. Another reason is that Kashmir is one of the leading fruit importing and exporting state, it is transported through trucks so truck drivers are also prone to this disease.
3. As for as females are concerned different surveys reveals that it security forces who forcefully rape at the time of cordon.

4. It has been observed that maximum numbers of case of HIV/AIDS were found in the 21-30 years age group as this is the sexually attractive age and very crucial stage.

CONCLUSION:

From the above discussion we can conclude that AIDS although a deadly disease, has not gone out of proportion in Kashmir. The limited number of cases reported so far is predominantly found among non locals. But that does not mean we should be complacent in tackling the disease given the fact that it could spread like fire in the forest. It would be appropriate to mention that AIDS in Kashmir is primarily spread through truck drivers, non- native laborers, and Security forces i.e. non-local sources. So such a mechanism should be developed which would effectively curtail import of HIV/AIDS into the state. Different but an important thing about HIV/AIDS in Kashmir, is that it is considered a taboo. People do not want to talk about it. Even those who are close to infected people- relatives and friends are looked down upon. All these things happen due to lack of proper knowledge about the disease. Government departments and institutions, Non Government Organizations and counseling centers should spread awareness about the disease with rejuvenated zeal.

REFERENCES

Aggarwal, V. (2008). Psychosocial aspects of people living with HIV/AIDS (PLHA). *Delhi psychiatry journal.* 11 (2). 174-176.

Basavarj, K.H., Navya, M.A. &Rashmi, R. (2010). Quality of life in HIV/AIDS. *Indian journal of sexually transmitted diseases and AIDS.* 31 (2). 75-80.

Bandawe, C.R. & Foster, D. (1996). AIDS-related beliefs, attitudes and intentions among
    Malawian students in three secondary schools. AIDS Care, 8(2), 223-232

Iqbal, M. (2015). HIV/AIDS and Social Exclusion in Kashmir. hyderabad, Telangana, india.
    IIPS/ORC Marco: National Family Health Survey of India 1998-99(2002). NFHS-2;

J& K, October, p. 149-55

Majumdar, B. &Mazaleni, N. (2010). The experiences of people living with HIV/AIDS and of their direct informal caregivers in a resource-poor setting. Journal of the international AIDS society. 13-20.

Revicki, D. A., Wu, A. W., & Murray, M. I. (1995). Change in clinical status, health status, and health utility outcomes in HIV-infected patients. Medical Care, 33(4), AS173-AS182.

Swindells, S., Mohr, J., Justis, J. C., Berman, S., Squier, C., Wagener, M. M., & Singh, N. (1999). Quality of life in patients with human immunodeficiency virus infection: Impact of social support, coping style and hopelessness. International Journal of STD & AIDS, 10, 383-391.

Wilson, H. S., Hutchinson, S. A., &Holzemer, W. L. (1997). Salvaging quality of life in ethnically diverse patients with advanced HIV/AIDS. Qualitative Health Research, 7, 75-87.

Wu, A. W., Matthews, W. C., Brysk, L. T. (1990). Quality of life in a placebo-controlled trial of zidovudine in patients with AIDS and AIDS-related complex. Journal of Acquired Immune Deficiency Syndromes, 5, 452-458.

Wu, A. W., Revicki, D. A., Jacobson, D., &Malitz, F. E. (1997). Evidence for the reliability, validity and usefulness of the Medical Outcomes Study HIV Health Survey (MOS-HIV). Quality of Life Research, 6, 481-493.

A Study of Stress & Anxiety in Pregnant Women: With Special Reference to their HIV Test

Dr. Krishna J. Vaghela[30]

ABSTRACT

The present study aimed to determine the difference of stress as well as anxiety among pregnant women in different age group with special reference to their HIV test. The present study recruited a sample of sixty pregnant women (30 pregnant women below 25 years and 30 pregnant women more than 35 years of age). All the participants were administered the stress measurement inventory and the anxiety scale. To obtained data were analyzed the interpreted using statistical tool such as men, standard deviation and the t-test. The results of the present study observed that there was no significant difference in stress as well as anxiety level of pregnant women before their HIV test. Both groups of pregnant women (age group of below 25 and more than 35 years of age) do not differ statistically significant on their level of stress as well as level of anxiety.

Keywords: *HIV-AIDS, HIV test, pregnant women, stress, anxiety*

The problem of HIV/AIDS is not only for underdeveloped countries but developing and developed countries are also faced this problem. Pregnancy is generally viewed as a common and positive event. Prior to 1994 there were few if any interventions known to reduce the risk of prenatal HIV transmission? However in 1994 the results of on American clinical trial known as ACTG 076 demonstrated that AZT administered to HIV positive pregnant women and to their children directly after birth could lower the rate of transmission from

---

[30] Associate, Professor & Head, Department of Psychology, Yogiji Maharaj Mahavidyalaya, Dhari, Dist. Amreli, (Gujarat)

25% to approximately 8%. Recent results appear to indicate that the actual rate of transmission can as low as 35% in many cases. These results are based on AZT administered to the woman during pregnancy, labour and delivery and to the newborn for the first six weeks of the life.

According to Selye (1956) any external event or internal drive which threatens to upset the orgasmic equilibrium is stress. Anxiety: 'A state of heightened emotional arousal containing a feeling of apprehension or dread like fear the subject feels threatened. Unlike fear, the subject often   perceives the source of the threat in vague or poorly defined terms.' 'Anxiety is a physiological state characterized by cognitive, somatic emotional and behavioral components.' Anxiety / stress disorders are a group of mental disorders.

 HIV is the virus that causes acquired immunodeficiency syndrome (AIDS) many women who have HIV do not know they are infected because it is possible to have HIV for years and not know it or not feel sick. A pregnant women need to HIV testing. If she has HIV in order to help for her and to reduce the risk of transmitting the infection to her baby.   About 0.2% (2of every 1000 women) of pregnant women are HIV positive of them about 1/3 (one out of every three) will pass the virus to their baby before it is born if no treatment is given. This is because the virus can cross to the baby from the mother's blood stream through the placenta as early as a woman's 8th week of pregnancy.

Stress is an inescapable part of modern life. Maternal stress affects the developing child before and after the birth. Before birth, severe and persistent glandular imbalance due to stress may result in irregularities in the developing child and complications are greater because the infant must often be delivered by instruments. Anxiety disorder is more likely to affect women than men and women who are pregnant are not excluded. In fact symptoms can develop or worsen during or after pregnancy though in some cases women notice fewer symptoms while pregnant.

Pregnant women experience a range of physical and emotional changes all of which may trigger anxiety. Researchers looked at the rates of detection and treatment of maternal anxiety by obstetricians during pregnancy and at six weeks postpartum. A further study focused on mothers older than 35, Lampine vehvilainem kanlkkunen (2009) from Finaland, reviewed women' altitude to the risk associated with pregnancy, in this maternal age group. They write, Being at risk (due to age) causes anxiety and concern which older pregnant women try to ease by preparing themselves for pregnancy and seeking information they receive can cause more anxiety rather than alleviate their concerns. Stress & anxiety during pregnancy has been associated with-increased risk of miscarriage, shorter gestation and higher incidence of preterm birth, smaller birth weight and length. The that maternal stress and anxiety during, pregnancy can have both immediate and long term effects on mother's (her) offspring.

HIV testing can be an emotional, stressful and anxious experience particularly for pregnant women. HIV testing was beneficial because it could help protect their babies from HIV infection. Routine testing does means that some woman will receive their diagnosis in pregnancy. For a newly diagnosed pregnant woman her HIV diagnosis is likely to be shocking and will provoke stress and anxiety. She will have concerns about her health, the health of her baby and the HIV status of her husband. To date insufficient studies have been conducted on the association between stress and anxiety during pregnancy and particular before HIV /AIDS test. Therefore the present study aims to reveal the difference of stress & anxiety among present women researching to their HIV test.

OBJECTIVES:-

- To study and compare the stress in pregnant women regarding to HIV test.
- To study and compare the anxiety in pregnant women regarding to HIV test.

Hypotheses:-

- There is no significant difference in stress level of pregnant women before their HIV test.
- There is no significant difference in anxiety level of pregnant women before their HIV test.
-

Procedure and participants:-

The present research recruited a sample of sixty participant's pregnant women. They come to different private clinics of Junagadh for their prenatal checkup. The present research conducted on a sample of sixty pregnant women among them thirty was below 25 years of age and thirty were more than 35 years of age. In the present sample included only those who had undergone pregnancy and were referred to HIV testing. Before their HIV testing the investigator requested them to participate in the study. The researcher used self administered questionnaires for collecting data. The questionnaires were given to pregnant women and they were requested to fill up them as per the instructions. No name were written on the questionnaires. Anonymity was maintained and participants were guaranteed confidentiality.

Measures:-

Following tools were used to collect the information.

Personal data sheet developed by investigator was used to collect some necessary information. To measure anxiety, Beck Anxiety Inventory was use. To measure stress, the stress measurement inventory developed by Bhatt was used. This inventory consists of 40 items. The reliability & validity to the test is 0.91 & 0.87.

Data analysis:-

The data obtained from the sample of sixty pregnant women were scored and analyzed. The analysis involved with mean, SD and t-test.

RESULTS AND DISCUSSION:-

The main purpose of the present study to examine the difference in stress as well as anxiety level of pregnant women regarding to their HIV test. For that purpose sixty pregnant women (age group of below 25 and more than 35 age) voluntarily participating in the present study. The following interpretation was made on the responses of sixty pregnant women with different age group. Ho-1, "there is no significant difference in stress level of pregnant women before their HIV test". The t-test was used to compare the score of stress of below 25 years and more than 35 years of age of pregnant women. The mean values of stress obtained by more than 35 years and below 25 years pregnant women's were 103.17 and 100.89 and the t-value was 1.17 which was not significant at 0.05 level of significance. The results indicated that there was statistically no significant difference on stress score of pregnant women. Therefore the null hypothesis was accepted and it clearly indicated that no significant difference was observed between comparative groups of pregnant women on their level of stress regarding to their HIV test.

Table-1, Mean, standard Deviation and t-test results comparing the pregnant women on stress.

Pregnant women age group	No.	Mean	S.D.	t-value	Sig.
More than 35	30	103.17	8.07	1.17	NS
Below 25	30	100.89	6.92		

Table-2, Mean, standard Deviation and t-test results comparing the pregnant women on anxiety.

Pregnant women age group	No.	Mean	S.D.	t-value	Sig.
More than 35	30	33.16	8.9	1.3	NS
Below 25	30	29.78	10.6		

The above table-2 indicates that there is no significant difference in the level of anxiety scores between the age group of below 25 and more than 35 years group of pregnant women. Therefore the null hypothesis: "there is no significant difference in anxiety level of pregnant women before their HIV test". It also accepted from table-2 it is observed that the mean value of anxiety score of more than 35 years age group pregnant women is 33.16 and below 25 years of age pregnant women is 29.78 and as the t-value (1.3) it found to be not significant. Thus it clearly indicates that the regarding the HIV test of pregnant women with different age group do not statistically significantly differ on their level of anxiety scores. Stress / anxiety during pregnancy can have long tern effects on the unborn child. HIV testing is recommended for all pregnant women. HIV can be passed from a mother to her baby during pregnancy, at delivery or during breast feeding. Mother's level of stress and anxiety may impact her baby. When a pregnant woman is stressed and experience anxiety the baby may be exposed to unhealthy levels of these hormones, which can impact the baby's brain development.

CONCLUSIONS:

The present study aims to reveal the difference of stress & anxiety among pregnant women regarding to their HIV test. After analysis and interpretation the following conclusions were drawn. There was no significant difference in stress level of pregnant women before their HIV test. As compare the anxiety level in pregnant women before their HIV test also statistically no significant difference was observed between age group of below 25 and more than 25 age group of pregnant women.

Acknowledgement:-

Thank the pregnant women who took part in present study for being generous with their time. Without them the study would not have been possible. I appreciate the staff at the gynecology clinics for their contribution in   the present study.

REFERENCES:

AIDS   Interventions in the Health Sector Progress Report 2010. Geneva; 2010.

 DSM III, Psychiatric Disorders in the United States, Results from the

Garret, H. E. (1971) Statistics in psychology and education, veils Feiffer and Simons

Kalpan, H.B. (1996) Psychological stress, New York : Academic press.

Kassler, R., Mc Gonagle, K., Zhao, S.(1994) Lifetime and 12 month prevalence of

Lampine, R, Vehvilainen, J. K. Kankkwnen, P. (2009) A Review of Pregnancy in Women over 35 years of age, The open Nursing Journal, Vol. -3, P. 3

National Co –Morbidity Survey, Arehigen Psychiatry 51, P.8 19.

National Guidelines on Prevention of Mother to Child Transmission of HIV in Nigeria.   4th ed. FMOH Abuja Nigeria: FMOH; 2010. P. - 113

 private ltd. 6th Indian addition Mumbai.

Shukla, K. C. (2005)   Encyclopedic dictionary of psychology, Commonwealth Publishers,   Ansari road, Darya Gang, New Delhi.

WHO, UNAIDS, Unicef: Towards Universal Access: Scaling up Priority HIV/

Anxiety among AIDS Patients: The Role of Age, Gender and Residence

Trupti Ambalal Chandalia[31], Dr. Hetal M. Patoliya[32]

ABSTRACT

The aim of the present study was to find out the difference in Anxiety with reference to age, gender and area of residence among AIDS patients. The participants were 360 AIDS patients was randomly selected from the Pandit Dindayal Upadhyay Government Hospital, ART center in the Rajkot city in Gujarat. The sample falls in the age range of 21-50 year. Anxiety scales constructed by Derogatis (1994) were used to measure Anxiety among AIDS patients. The data was analysedusing 'F' test and tukey test. The result revealed significant difference in anxiety between male and female AIDS patients. It was observed that the female had high anxiety than male AIDS patients, area group no difference and old age high anxiety than young age AIDS patients.

Keywords: HIV-AIDS, Anxiety and AIDS Patients.

The human immunodeficiency virus (HIV) is an infectious disease that compromises the human immune system, allowing opportunistic infections and cancers that would otherwise be easily suppressed, to thrive. HIV is transmitted by bodily fluids (Blood, semen) and can go undetected in individuals for years before AIDS-defining illnesses appear (Gandhi, Skanderson, Gordon, Concato, & Justice, 2007). Today the HIV virus and its progression to acquired immunodeficiency syndrome (AIDS) is recognized as a worldwide pandemic by the World Health Organization (UNAIDS & WHO, 2007). Over 33 million individuals are currently infected and the disease is estimated to be responsible for approximately 2 million

---
[31] Research Fellow, Department of Psychology, Saurashtra University, Rajkot
[32] Assistant Professor, Department of Psychology, Saurashtra University, Rajkot

deaths annually (UNAIDS & WHO, 2007). Although in the United States HIV/AIDS once primarily affected White gay and bisexual men (Kelly & Murphy, 1992), it is now increasingly more common among heterosexual men and individuals in minority ethnic groups (CDC, 2008). Estimates from 33 states with long-term, confidential name-based HIV/AIDS databases indicate that there are approximately one million two hundred thousand individuals living with HIV/AIDS in the United States today (CDC, 20012).

There are an estimated 4.2 million people living with HIV in Asia, 90% of them are in India, China and Thailand. India contributes 49% of it (2.4 million people). The first focuses of HIV in India were detected in 1986 among sex workers in Chennai and the first AIDS case was reported in 1987 in Mumbai. Like in other countries, HIV was accompanied with stigma, discrimination, depression, suicidal tendencies and violence. Right from the beginning of the epidemic in India, an AIDS task force was established by the Indian Council of Medical Research (ICMR) for screening risk behaviour of such groups. As more cases began to be detected, a National AIDS Committee was set up under the Union Ministry of Health and Family Welfare in 1986. The objective of this committee was to control the spread of the infection and promote community and family-based care to people with HIV/AIDS. The National AIDS Control Organization (NACO) was established in 1992 and the first National AIDS Control Programme (NACP) was launched. Its main objective at that time was to undertake surveillance to know modes of spread, to screen blood and increase awareness. By early 1990s, cases of HIV infection had been reported in every state of the country and it was clear that individual states had different prevalence rates. In 1998, 176 surveillance sites were established and a nationwide surveillance was done, which revealed that there might be nearly 3 million HIV-infected persons in India

Despite the availability of effective cognitive and pharmaceutical treatments, anxiety remains one of the most commonly diagnosed mental health conditions affecting persons living with human immunodeficiency virus (HIV) disease (Bing et al. 2001; Whetten et al. 2008). Many aspects of HIV disease create potential for generating anxiety including financial difficulties, limited access to care, encountering HIV stigma, disclosure concerns, symptoms associated with HIV disease progression and an uncertain disease course (Lee et al. 2002). Anxiety symptoms also impact health outcomes in HIV disease. They are strong predictors of non-adherence with HIV medications and, as a result, anxiety symptoms may hasten HIV disease progression (Campos et al. 2010). They can also contribute to a diminished quality of life as well as higher costs of health care (Ford et al. 2004). Along with a growing body of research directed towards the testing of psychosocial clinical interventions for HIV-related anxiety, there has been a continuing interest in developing self management strategies for coping with anxiety symptoms.

A growing body of research presents evidence of the high prevalence of anxiety disorders among persons living with HIV disease (Bing et al. 2001; Kemppainen et al. 2006; Whetten et al. 2008). Prevalence rates of anxiety disorders have been estimated to be as high as 38%, compared to 11% in the general population (Pence et al. 2007). In addition to increased rates of generalized anxiety disorder and panic disorder, studies also reflect high rates of post-traumatic stress disorder (PTSD; O'Cleirigh et al. 2009; Reisner et al. 2009). Multiple investigators suggest that anxiety disorders may be highest among groups with the highest HIV prevalence rates including high-risk women of colour and men who have sex with men (O'Cleirigh et al. 2009). Studies also highlight the co-occurrence of HIV-related anxiety with other mental health disorders, including substance use and mood disorders (Gaynes et al. 2008).

Psychological disorders like depression and anxiety are potentially dangerous conditions, in the context of HIV/AIDS, which can influence health-seeking behaviour or uptake of diagnosis and treatment for HIV/AIDS. More recent research demonstrates a linkage between anxiety and adverse physiological changes in HIV. Increased levels of psychological distress, including anxiety, may result in the deregulation of stress regulation hormones, a diminished regulation of the immune system, an impaired response to HIV medications (Greeson et al. 2008; Lampe et al. 2010) and increased severity of fatigue (Barroso et al. 2010). Looking at this aspect the present study was carried out with following objectives:

OBJECTIVES

1. To find out the difference in anxiety between female and male AIDS patients.
2. To find out the difference in anxiety between rural and urban area AIDS patients.
3. To find out the difference in anxiety between young age and old age AIDS patients.

METHOD

Sample:

The sample for the present study consisted of 180 female and 180 male AIDS patients were selected randomly from Pandit Dindayal Upadhyay Government Hospital, Antiviral Therapy (ART) Rajkot city in Gujarat. The age range of students was 21-50 year AIDS patients.

Tool:

The following tools were used in the present study:

1. Personal Data Sheet:

Personal data sheet was prepared to collect some personal information such as age, gender, family income, area type etc.

2. Anxiety Scale (SCL-90-R Scale):

This 90-item self-report symptom inventory measures a broad range of psychological problems and symptoms through nine primary symptom dimensions including somatization, obsession-compulsion, interpersonal sensitivity, depression, anxiety, hostility, phobic anxiety, paranoid ideation and psychoticism (Derogatis et al. 1973). The SCL-90 is designed for use with individuals from the community as well as persons with medical or psychiatric conditions. The SCL-90 is scored on a five-point scale assessing 'how much' the respondent was bothered by each symptom in the past week (0 = not at all; 4 = extremely). The instrument has well-established reliability and validity and has been tested across numerous populations 13 years old and older (Derogatis & Unger 2010). In this study, anxiety symptoms were assessed with the 10-item anxiety subscale from the SCL-90. The items in this subscale are summed to obtain a total score that can range from 0 to 40. Internal consistency in this sample was high (Cronbach's $\alpha = 0.95$).

Procedure:

The investigation explained the purpose of the study to the subjects. When the subject was comfortable with instructions and ready for testing, questionnaires were given. They were asked to answer each and every item of all the administered questionnaires and were ensured that the responses given by them would be kept confidential. Scoring was carried out as per the manual. F test and Tukey test was used for statistical analysis.

RESULT AND DISCUSSION

In order to objectives of the study data were analyzed using F-test. When the statistical analysis regarding the impact of use of gender, area of residence and age on anxiety among AIDS patients was carried out interesting results were obtained. These results are presented in above tables.

Table-1, ANOVA summary of Anxiety with reference to gander, area and age to AIDS patients

Source	S. S.	df	M. S.	F
A (Gander)	525.63	1	525.63	20.63[**]
B (Area)	0.23	1	0.23	0.009[NS]
C (Age)	309.51	2	154.75	6.08[**]
ABSS	166.74	1	166.75	6.55[**]
ACSS	285.72	2	142.86	5.61[**]
BCSS	102.05	2	51.03	2.01[NS]
ABCSS	99.37	2	49.69	1.95[NS]
WSS	8856.43	348	25.45	
TSS	10345.66	359		

**=P<0.01, NS=Not Significant

As gender was one of the factors included in factorial design 2x2x3 ANOVA carried out and the F-Value (Table-1) was found to be 20.63which is significant at 0.01 level. Thus, the result revealed significant impact of gander on anxiety among AIDS patients. Reveals that the mean scores of anxiety of female and male are 21.34 and 19.32 respectively difference of the mean 2.02 is remarkable. Concluded the female had high anxiety than male AIDS patients. The results in regard to the main effect of gender clearly indicated that HIV positive females had greater scores on composite anxiety and its feeling component than male counterparts. The findings are, therefore, consistent with those reported by Larson and Pleck (1999) and Barroso, Carlson, and Meynell (2003).The result of the present study is supported by other studies (Ashmore, 1990; Brody & Holly, 1999; Martinez et. al., 2002 and Prentiss et. al., 2007). The probable reason for this difference Taylor (2006) also reports that as HIV positive women suffer from critical gynaecological infections too, mere counselling seems to produce less effect on them as compared to male patients. It is, therefore, suggested that counselling needs to be combined with some other therapeutic procedure to relieve the female patients from anxiety to a greater extent. suggested that counselling needs to be combined with some other therapeutic procedure to relieve the female patients from anxiety to a greater extent.

When F-test was applied to examine to impact of residence area on AIDS patients not significant impact was found. The F- value is 0.009 which is no significant Reveals that the mean scores of anxiety of rural and urban AIDS patients are 20.56 and 20.51 respectively no significant difference of the mean 0.05.

When F-test was applied to examine to impact of age on AIDS patients significant impact was found. The F- value is 6.08 which are significant at 0.01 level. Thus, the result revealed significant impact of age on anxiety among AIDS patients. Reveals that the mean scores of anxiety of 21 year to 30 year, 31 year to 40 year and 41 year to 50 year are 20.01, 19.75 and 21.85 respectively difference of the mean (C_1 vs C_2) 0.26, (C_1 vs C_3) 1.84 and (C_2 vs C_3) 2.10 is remarkable. Concluded the female had high anxiety than male AIDS patients.

Table-2, Tukey test summary for Anxiety with reference to gander, area and age group

Groups	C_1	C_2	C_3
20.01	-	0.26^{NS}	1.84^{*}
19.75	-	-	2.10^{**}
21.83	-	-	-

*P<0.05, **P<0.01, NS= Not Significant

Groups	A2B1	A2B2	A1B2	A1B1
18.67	-	1.31^{NS}	2.36^{**}	3.78^{**}
19.98	-	-	1.05^{NS}	2.47^{**}
21.03	-	-	-	1.42^{NS}
22.45	-	-	-	-

**P<0.01, NS= Not Significant

Groups	A2C1	A2C3	A2C2	A1C2	A1C1	A1C3
18.65	-	0.97	1.05	1.15	2.72	5.40
19.62	-	-	0.08	0.18	1.75	4.43
19.70	-	-	-	0.10	1.67	4.35
19.80	-	-	-	-	1.57	4.25
21.37	-	-	-	-	-	2.68
24.05	-	-	-	-	-	-

**P<0.01, NS= Not Significant

So far as the impact of age on AIDS patients is concerned out of possible three comparisons two mean differences were found significant at 0.01 and 0.05 level by computing Tukey test. The most striking results were obtained for the group of AIDS patients with old age group. This group of AIDS patients significantly differed with group of AIDS patients with C_1 vs C_3 and C_2 vs C_3 age groups. Thus, AIDS patients with 41 to 50 year age group experienced high anxiety and AIDS patients with 20 to 31 year age group indicate low anxiety. The result of the present study is supported by other studies (Israelski Gore Feltoen, Power, Wood and Koopman, 2001).

So far as the impact of gander and area on anxiety is concerned, results of Post hoc Tukey test revealed that out of possible six comparisons three mean differences were found significant at 0.01 level. The most striking results were obtained for the group of AIDS patients with female at rural area group and AIDS patients with male at urban area group indicate low anxiety.

So far as the impact of gander, area and age on anxiety is concerned, results of Post hoc Tukey test revealed that out of possible fifteen comparisons six mean differences were found significant at 0.01 level. The most striking results were obtained for the group of AIDS patients with 41 to 50 year age of female group and AIDS patients with 41 to 50 year age of male group indicate low anxiety.

CONCLUSION

As far as gender is concerned gender and age group significantly differenced in anxiety, that means female AIDS patients are high on anxiety than male AIDS patients and area of residence group is no significant difference. As far as age group is concerned old age AIDS patients are significantly anxiety than young age AIDS patients.

REFERENCE

Ashmore MC 1990. Entrepreneurship in vocational education. In: Kent CA. (ed.). *Entrepreneurship education: current developments, future directions*. New York: Quorum Books.

Barroso, J., Carlson, J. R., & Meynell,J. (2003). Physiological and psychological markers associated with HIV-related fatigue. *Clinical Nursing Research, 12*(1), 49-68.

Barroso, J., et al. (2010) Physiological and psychological factors that predictHIV-related fatigue. *AIDS and Behavior*, **14** (6), 1415–1427.

Bing, E.G., Burnam, M.A. & Longshore, D. (2001) Psychiatric disorders and drug use among human immunodeficiency virus-infected adults in the United States. *Archives of General Psychiatry*, **58**, 721–728.

Brody GH. Sibling relationship quail ty: Its causes and consequences. Annual Review of Psychology 1998;49:1-24.

Campos, L., Guimares, M. & Reimen, R. (2010) Anxiety and depression symptoms as risk factors for non-adherence to antiretroviral therapies in Brazil. *AIDS and Behavior*, **14** (2), 289–299.

Center for Disease Control and Prevention (2012). *HIV in the United States at a Glance.*

Center for Disease Control and Prevention. (2008). *Estimates of new HIV infections in the United States.*

Derogatis LR, Lipman RS & Covi C (1973) SCL-90: an outpatient psychiatric rating scale preliminary report. Psychopharmacol Bull 9: 13 27.

Ford, J., et al. (2004) Prospective association of anxiety, depression, and addictive disorders with high utilization of primary, specialty, and emergency medical care. *Social Science and Medicine*, **58**, 2145–2148.

Gandhi, N. R., Skanderson, M., Gordon, K. S., Concato, J., & Justice, A. C. (2007). Delayed presentation for human immunodeficiency virus (HIV) care among veterans: A problem of access or screening? *Medical Care, 45*(11), 1105-1109. doi:10.1097/MLR.0b013e3181271476

Gaynes, B.N., Pence, B.W., Eron, J.J. & Miller,W.C. (2008) Prevalence and co morbidity of psychiatric diagnoses based on reference standard in an HIV+ patient population. *Psychosomatic Medicine,* **70**, 505–511.

Greeson, J.M., et al. (2008) Psychological distress, killer lymphocytes and disease severity in HIV/AIDS. *Brain Behavior, and Immune,* **6**, 901– 911.

Ham, V. et al. (2002), ―What makes for effective teacher professional development in ICT?,‖ EducationCounts.[Online].Available:

Israelski E.W., and W.H.Muto. (2007) "Human Factors Risk Management in Medical Products" Handbook of Human Factors and Ergonomics in Health Care and Patient Safety. P Carayon, ed. Lawrence Erlbaum Associates: Mahwah, NJ.

Kemppainen, J., et al. (2006) Strategies for self-management of HIV-related anxiety. *AIDS Care,* **18** (6), 597–607.

Lampe, F., et al. (2010) Physical and psychological symptoms and risk of virologic rebound among patients with virologic suppression on antiretroviral therapy. *Journal of Acquired Immune Deficiency Syndrome,* **54** (5), 500–505.

Larson, R., & Pleck, J. (1999). Hidden feelings: Emotionality in boys and girls. In D. Bernstein (Ed.), *Gender and Motivation* (Vol. 45, pp. 25-74). Lincoln: University of Nebraska Press.

Lee, R., Kochman, A. & Sikkema, K. (2002) Internalized stigma among people living with HIV/AIDS. *AIDS and Behavior,* **6** (4), 309–319.

Martinez, C., M. Michaud, R.R. Bélanger, and R.J. Tweddell. 2002. Identification of soils suppressive against Helminthosporium solani , the causal agent of potato silver scurf. Soil Biol. Biochem. 34 : 1861-1868.

NACO website, 'About NACO, National AIDS Control Programme Phase 1 (1992-1999)', accessed 4/7/06

O'Cleirigh, C., Skeer, M., Mayer, K. & Safren, S. (2009) Functional impairment and health care utilization among HIV-infected men who have sex with men: the relationship with depression and post-traumatic stress. *Journal of Behavioral Medicine,* **32** (5), 466–477.

Prentiss, Anna Marie, Natasha Lyons, Lucille E. Harris, Melisse R.P. Burns, Terrence M. Godin. 2007. The emergence of status inequality in intermediate scale societies: A demographic and socio- economic history of the Keatley Creek site, British Columbia. Journal of Anthropological Archaeology26: 299–327.

Reisner, S., Mimiaga, M., Safren, S. & Mayer, K. (2009) Stressful or traumatic life events, post-traumatic stress disorder (PTSD) symptoms, and HIV sexual risk taking among men who have sex with men. *AIDS Care*, **21** (12), 1481–1489.

Taylor, S. E. (2006). *Health Psychology*. New Delhi: Tata McGraw Hill.

Whetten, K., Reif, S.,Whetten, R. & Murphy-McMillan, L. (2008) Trauma, mental health, distrust, and stigma among HIV-positive persons: implications for effective care. *Psychosomatic Medicine*, **70** (5), 531–538.

WHO (2008). HIV/AIDS and mental health. Geneva, Switzerland: WHO.

World Health Organization, UNAIDS, UNICEF. *Towards universal access: scaling up priority HIV/AIDS interventions in the health sector: progress report.* April 2007. Geneva: WHO.

Impact of Geographical Locale and Education on the Awareness towards HIV/AIDS among Adolescents

Urvashi Singh[33], Shalini Singh[34]

ABSTRACT

The main emphasis of the present research was to study the impact of locale and education on the awareness towards HIV/AIDS among adolescent group. The sample comprised of 300 adolescents belonging to an age group of 15-17 years. 150 adolescents belonged to rural group and 150 belonged to urban group. On the other hand 150 were educated up to senior secondary level while 150 were educated up to graduation level. The entire sample was of the male adolescents. A checklist was prepared that was named as HIV (AIDS) Awareness questionnaire. It dealt with various issues like social mobility, social support, healthiness, well-being, role of media etc. in curbing this stigma. The data was analyzed through ANOVA which indicated that level of Education and Geographical locale had significant impact on the awareness towards HIV/AIDS in our youth.

Keywords: HIV-AIDS, Education, Awareness, Locale, Healthiness, social support

The Human Immunodeficiency Virus (HIV) is the virus that causes HIV infection. When infected, the virus replicates and can attack the infection-fighting T-cells of the body's immune system. Loss of t-cells makes it difficult for immune system to fight infections. If left untreated, HIV can progress and cause Acquired Immunodeficiency Syndrome (AIDS). Globally, almost of a quarter of people living with Human Immunodeficiency Virus (HIV) are under the age of 25 years (UNAIDS, 2004). In India, 35 % of all reported AIDS cases

---

[33] Asst. Professor, Draunacharya College, Gurgaon
[34] Professor, Dept. of Psychology, MDU Rohtak

are among the age group of 15-24 years, indicating the vulnerability of the younger population to epidemic (National AIDS control organization, 2005). Furthermore, the epidemic is moving from high risk groups such as sex workers to the general population and from Urban to rural population (Park, 2007). We can contract HIV through mutual blood or semen contract. This most often occurs during unprotected sex or by sharing needles during injection drug use. There are also cases where a mother passes the virus on to the newborn or transmits the virus via breastfeeding. HIV/AIDS places an increasing burden on the health of the population, and cause further socio-economic problems for individuals, families, communities and governments in many countries. (Beck et al: 2001 & Walker et al. 2004). HIV affects the immune system and reduces the body's defenses to protect against various infectious diseases and cancer. Treatment is available to delay the death of person suffering from disease; however there is no cure. Thus it becomes necessary to educate young people so that they can protect themselves from getting infected. In 2009 alone, there were 890,000 new HIV infections amongst young people aged 15-24 (UNAIDS/UNICEF, 2010) and in 2010,5 million 15-24 years old were living with HIV (WHO/UNAIDS/UNICEF, 2012). If somebody has been tested positive for HIV, then one should immediately meet HIV specialist as soon as possible. There are tests that can be done if it is progressing. For this, anti-HIV medication regimen is to be started and start working towards an undetectable viral load. Antiretroviral Therapy (ART) is the recommended treatment for HIV infection. To stop the spread of HIV/AIDS various government and non government organizations in the world over have undertaken programs to raise awareness and among people regarding HIV/AIDS. Quinn and Overbaugh, (2005) found that India has emerged as major player in the global HIV epidemic and has given the importance of adolescents in Indian epidemic. The lack of information on knowledge, perceptions and behaviors regarding HIV and preventing behaviors among Indian adolescents are found important factors and need to be pondered over.

OBJECTIVES

- There would be significant effect of locale on the awareness towards HIV/AIDS among adolescents.
- There would be significant effect of level of education on awareness towards HIV/AIDS among adolescents.

METHOD

Design:

It was a 2×2 factorial design study. There were two independent variables, i.e. level of education and geographical locale. The first variable was varied at two levels, i.e. senior secondary (12th class) and graduation level. The second independent variable was locale that also dealt at two levels, i.e. urban and rural. The end variable was awareness towards HIV/AIDS.

Sample:

The sample comprised of 300 male adolescents belonging to an age group of 15-17 years. 150 subjects were taken from urban background. 150 subjects were taken from rural background. In each group there were 150 were educated up to Senior Secondary while in another group 150 were educated up to graduation level.

Tools:

A checklist was prepared of 30 items dealing with factors responsible for HIV/AIDS, awareness paradigm and coping strategies to overcome this stigma. It also included some of health issues, i.e. healthiness, resilience, optimism etc. The basic impetus of this checklist was to assess the awareness towards HIV/AIDS. It was on 4 point ratings scale; as the higher the score higher is awareness.

RESULT AND DISCUSSION:

Table no. 1 clearly reveals the ANOVA for HIV/AIDS awareness and mean score are depicted in table no. 2 and table no. 3.

Table 1: summary for ANOVA for HIV/AIDS Awareness

Square of variance	Ss	df	Ms	F
A(I)	1725.20	1	315.29	75.40**
B(II)	1020.25	1	220.25	24.79**
A×B	15.86	1	7.24	.89
Within Group	1899.19	296	10.24	

Table No. 1clearly reveals the F value for locale is 75.40, p<.01 which is significant. Further the F value for level of education is 24.79, p<.01 which is also significant. It means that urban adolescents with higher educational level have more awareness of HIV/AIDS.

Table 2: Mean Scores of HIV/AIDS Awareness for factor-I (A: Locale)

A(Locale)	N	Total	Mean
A_1(Urban)	150	17250	105
A_2(Rural)	150	9000	60

Table No. 2 clearly reveals that the adolescents belonging to urban areas had much higher mean scores regarding the awareness of HIV/AIDS i.e. mean 105. While the rural subjects had very low mean scores, i.e. 60 clearly denoting lack of awareness about this menace. It is because urban adolescents have more exposure and knowledge about the various issues prevailing in society. These may vary from various social problems to illness to epidemics.

Table 3: Mean Scores of HIV/AIDS Awareness for factor B (II) (Level of Education)

B(Level of Education)	N	Total	Mean
B$_1$ (Graduate)	150	15000	100
B$_2$ (Senior Secondary)	150	9000	60

Table No. 3 clearly shows the higher awareness scores about HIV in those subjects who are graduate than those who are just educated up to senior secondary level. The rationale behind these findings clearly show that more educated people have more updated knowledge, better opportunities to grow and develop and at the same time have high awareness to remain hale, healthy and illness free. On the other hand, those adolescents who are not well-read need to make aware about this serious infectious disease.

The need of an hour requires various interventions to create awareness:-

- To observe world AIDS day (Dec. I) in every educational institute belonging to any area whether rural, semi-rural or urban.
- Try to impart sex education to students at school level after fifth standard.
- Youth Risk Behavior Surveillance System for 9th to 12th Grade students should be monitored.
- Since rate of HIV infections vary significantly in lower income communities and semi-urban area, government and non government organizations should make such programmes where they can educate the youth about health care , stigma and discrimination, as well as a prevalence of unrecognized and untreated infectious that allow the virus to spread.

- Time to time life skill workshops and conferences should be organized in schools and community to be more aware, awaken and away from this serious problem.

REFERENCES

Beck, E.J, Miners, A.H, & Tolley, K. (2001). The cost of HIV treatment and care: a global review, Pharmacoeconomics, 19: 13-39.

Park, K. (2007). AIDS. In Park K, editor. Textbook of Preventive and social Medicine, 19th edition, Jabalpur Banarasidas Bhanot. 285-297.

Quinn, T.C. and Overbaugh, J. (2005). HIV/AIDS in women: an expanding epidemic, Science, 308:5728, 1582-1583.

UNAIDS Inter-agency Task Team on Young People (2004) At the crossroads: Accelerating Youth Access to HIV/AIDS Interventions UNAIDS New York, Retrieved from http://www.unfpa.org/upload/lib_pub_file//316_filename-UNFPA-Crossroads.pdf. On 12.03.2014

Walker, N. Grassly, N.C. Garnett, G.P. Stanecki, K.A. Ghys, P.D. (2004). Estimating the global burden of HIV/AIDS: what do we really know about the HIV Pandemic? Lancet; 363: 2180-5. 10.

Family Adjustment, Social Adjustment and Depression in People with HIV Positive Diagnosis

Dr. Ashokbhai J. Gohil[35], Vishal P. Parmar[36]

ABSTRACT

The present research focuses on individuals suffering from HIV positive diagnosis. The study aims to understand the level of family and social adjustment and levels of depression in these people. For the same purpose, a sample of 240 individuals were selected from Ahmedabad and Bhavnagar regions out of them 120 (60 male and 60 female) were from Urban and 120 (60 male and 60 female) were from Rural area individuals who were suffering from HIV positive diagnosis. Gujarati adaptation of Bail adjustment inventory by Dr. D.J Bhatt and Chauhan and Tiwari's depression scale was used for assessment. The data was analysed using 't' test. Results indicate that there are better adjustment levels in family and social aspects and reduced levels of depression after counselling.

Keywords: *HIV-AIDS, Family Adjustment, Social Adjustment, Depression, Urban, Rural, Male, Female*

Human Immunodeficiency Virus or Acquired Immune Deficiency Syndrome (HIV/AIDS) is a broad spectrum of conditions which is caused by being infected from HIV. Following the infection, a number of symptoms are experienced by the individual which interferes with his/her physical and mental health to a great extent. HIV/AIDS is a well known condition and has affected large number of people since its discovery. With the increasing number of people being diagnosed with this condition, there are also rising

---

[35] Laboratory Technician, Forensic Psychology Division, DFS, Gandhinagar

[36] M.phil Forensic Psychology Trainee , Institute of Behavioural Science (IBS), Gujarat Forensic Sciences University, Gandhinagar, Gujarat

misunderstandings regarding the nature of the disease. In such a scenario, an individual with HIV positive diagnosis has a tough battle to fight. It becomes difficult to create and maintain an environment which is respects equality and fairness. Not only this, it is also important that the families of such individuals are aware about their condition and are willingly providing care to them and supporting them to live in the society at large. Care needs to be taken in a manner in which even unknowingly the individual is not hurt.

Apart from making everyday changes and adjustments to live a better life, there are many other aspects in the life of an individual with HIV/AIDS diagnosis which need to be highlighted. Thoughts about the illness, physical symptoms, social stigma, acceptance from family, fear of death and various other questions keep running in their minds. Such thoughts and feelings lead to experiencing sad mood and feeling lost. Thus, constant support from immediate family members and professional help from counsellors is important.

In India, HIV/AIDS infection had been seen as a serious illness from the beginning itself. Initial cases included working women in Chennai and Mumbai being infected by using injection needles. Soon, the disease started spreading to other parts of the country at a rapid pace, infecting many other individuals. Newer cases started getting recorded as infection spread from urban to smaller rural regions, wherein the situation was more critical as rural people were more vulnerable to the disease. Recent researches have shown that pregnant women out of all the recorded cases of HIV/AIDS, 90% fall into the age group of 18-40 years which is also considered to be that age group which falls into the earning population. Thus, affecting the overall economy of the country on a large level. When a family member of this age group, gets infected with the disease, it affects the total family income, creating disputes and straining their relationships. These families also face an added burden of pooling in money for the treatment of the individual as he/she keeps falling ill time and again and needs regular medications. Such issues put these families into financial difficulties and create an environment of worry for the HIV/AIDS patient as well. It could also be a possibility that the patient's workplace does not have a positive attitude towards him/her and towards the illness for e.g. avoiding the patient, staying away from him/her, not willing to work with him/her, etc. Close friends and relatives also tend to change their behaviour towards the patient, thus creating a socially isolated environment wherein it becomes difficult for the patient to express his/her needs and reduces the adjustment level in society. Due to such issues, the present study focuses on the importance of consistent counselling for patients suffering from HIV/AIDS.

Counselling for HIV/AIDS patients

Since HIV/AIDS is a disease which comes with various issues including health concerns, social stigma, unemployment, attitude of family members and much more, it becomes extremely important for these patients to undergo counselling on a regular basis. The individual may be having negative thoughts related to his/her health, fear of not being accepted, losing his/her social ties, misperceptions regarding the illness, worry, fear of dying among others. When counselling for such issues is given, the person feels connected to another being that tries and understands his/her perspective and helps him/her find a way to cope. It also helps in increasing one's self confidence and provides more courage to live and fight the battle. One very important goal achieved through counselling is of providing details about the illness to the individual. Many a times not being aware regarding what is happening with our body creates panic in many patients. Thus, it provides relief to know what is happening at present, how he/she got infected, what could be the possible consequences and how he/she should prepare self for the same and others. Counselling is also a process wherein the patient can comfortably share his fears. Since HIV/AIDS is a disease which affects many areas of one's life, small everyday matters which may seem simple to others, may become a matter of worry for the patient. Thus, counselling is essential.

Different stages have different counselling procedures which need to be followed. Pre-test counselling is provided to those individuals who want to give their blood samples for testing. Post-test counselling is required by individuals who have already undergone the testing procedure and are waiting for the reports or have already received the reports and need advice for the same. Drug adherence counselling makes the patients understand the importance of medication in order to cope with the disease and consequences of skipping doses or terminating medicines without consultation with the doctor.

Adjustment

Adjustment is an important part of life. According to Boring Lang Field, adjustment is an act through which an individual tries to maintain a balance between his needs and factors which will help him fulfil those needs. In simple words it could be defined as learning to make changes in our behaviour according to the situation in which we are placed. Humans are social beings and thus adjustment is required the most in our lives as we need to maintain a certain level of comfort with friends, family, colleagues, relatives, neighbours and others in order to work and live in a harmonious manner. A person living with HIV/AIDS may have difficulty adjusting in many areas of life. There are many misconceptions regarding the disease and thus it may be that the individual remains being misunderstood by others. If others do not show understanding and acceptance to the patient, he/she may feel neglected and misunderstood and hence is not able to make adjustments.

Family Adjustment:

Though members of a family are close to each other, at times there are moments wherein adjusting within family is not easy. HIV/AIDS patient may face this situation more often as they may feel weak due to their poor health conditions and not being able to contribute financially for the family. Worry keeps developing regarding the economical condition of the family. Moreover, at times family members may behave indifferently towards the patient, or do not accept the patient and his/her condition thus making it more difficult for the patient to adjust. Due to wrong information about the disease, there might be some behaviour on the part of the family which may hurt the patient for e.g. keeping the patient's bed separate, using different utensils for the patient, etc. Such behaviours break the patient mentally and makes adjustment a difficult job.

Social Adjustment:

Since humans need other human beings to maintain a social environment around them, it is important that one learns how to make social adjustments. When we talk about social relationships, we not only include relations with family, friends, colleagues and others but also includes society at large. Thus, it becomes important to define what we call as a society. According to Right, society is not just a cluster of human beings living together. Rather it is an arrangement in which social relationships between human beings keep developing. There are a lot indifference faced by the person suffering from HIV/AIDS for e.g. being neglected by friends and colleagues at workplace. Such social isolation from important individuals in the patient's life make it difficult for him to develop and maintain social relationships and thus make him/her social isolated. By living in the society, our physical and mental needs are understood and fulfilled by others and the same is reciprocated by us. Any relationship is based on the 'give and take' phenomenon. We receive what we give. Relationships come with certain responsibilities which need to be fulfilled by us but at times this is not possible. This many a times hurts us and creates discomfort in relations. HIV/AIDS patient may or may not have social ties as it may become difficult for him/her to fulfil such responsibilities all the time. They need people who understand them and their condition in its correct form. Misinformed people can do more harm than good to these patients.

Depression

Adjustment in life is necessary but unfortunately it is not something that we can do all the time and hence has certain consequences which we need to face. Depression is one such consequence. When one is not able to make adjustments, need fulfilment gets blocked and this leads to the feeling of being depressed and the person undergoes a lot of mental conflict. A depressed person cannot fight the odds that he/she is facing and thus feels that things are getting out of control. Morgan defines depression as any situation wherein a person's needs are not fulfilled in a given timeframe. Anything which delays need gratification can lead to feeling depressed.

Various symptoms in a person can help us identify whether he/she is going through depression or not. These symptoms are divided into physical symptoms and psychological symptoms. Physical symptoms include dry mouth, decreased appetite and sleep, decreased energy, feeling tired, lazy, irritable mood, downward gaze, low speech tone, may have respiratory problems and may develop substance use. Psychological symptoms include worthlessness, hopelessness, decreased self confidence, worry, fearful, not finding happiness or enjoyment in daily activities, social withdrawal, feelings of failure, confusion, indecisiveness, losing meaning from life, self blaming and suicidal ideations or plans of attempt.

Individuals suffering from HIV/AIDS have enough reasons to undergo depression. Concerns regarding health, financial conditions, interpersonal relations, attitude of family members, acceptance level, blaming self for contracting the disease and many other aspects create negative thoughts and later lead to depressive feelings. They undergo a lot of stressful situations and thus may remain confused as

232

they are not able to come to any conclusion. In such circumstances, a positive and accepting environment from the family, sufficient moral support and professional help from a counsellor can make life a little better for the patients.

OBJECTIVE

The major objectives of the study are:
1. To know the level of family Adjustment of HIV positive people before and after counseling.
2. To know the level of Social Adjustment of HIV positive people before and after counseling.
3. To know the level of Depression of HIV positive people before and after counseling.

Hypothesis

Hypothesis is considered as the principal instrument in research (Khothari, 1990). Any research starts with hypothesis. So hypothesis is such a factor that its reliability remains to be checked. In this study, the following null hypotheses which will be tested.

The present study was undertaken with the following

Ho_1: There will be no significant difference in level of Family Adjustment in HIV positive people in relation to before and after Counseling.

Ho_2: There will be no significant difference in level of Social Adjustment in HIV positive people in relation to before and after Counseling.

Ho_3: There will be no significant difference in level of Depression in HIV positive people in relation to before and after Counseling.

METHOD

Sample

After finalizing the variables of the present study, consideration was given to whether the entire population for being the subjects for data collection or a particular group was to be selected as a representative of the whole population. For this research we selected those cities that have community care centres. Finally all data of HIV positive people were collected from Ahmedabad and Bhavnagar City. Total 240 HIV positive people were selected as a sample which comprised of 120 male and 120 females.

Sample (240)

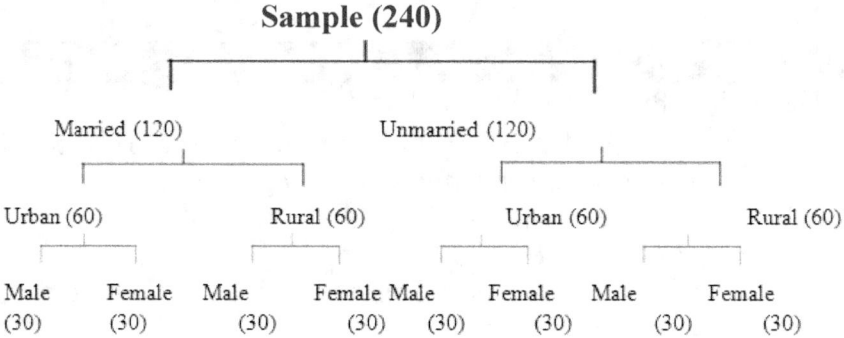

The selected respondents constitute is technically called a sample. (Khothari, 1990). In the present research parents of HIV positive people 120 people were selected from Urban and 120 people were selected from rural area of Gujarat State.

Tool

1. Bail adjustment inventory

Gujarati adaptation of Bail adjustment inventory by Dr. D.J Bhatt was used to measure adjustment level of HIV Positive people. Here we used two adjustment inventories from it:

     1. Family adjustment inventory

     2. Social adjustment inventory

Statistical properties of the inventory: The test-retest reliability is 0.76 and half-split reliability is 0.87. For the family adjustment inventory reliability is 0.78 and for the social adjustment inventory it is 0.76. Test-retest time duration was 30 days.

2. Depression scale

Prof N.S Chauhan and Govind Tiwari's Depression Scale Was used to know the level of Depression in HIV Positive people. It is a 5 point scale with total 40 sentence form items.

Statistical properties of the scale: The test-retest reliability of this scale is 0.79 and split half reliability is 0.76. The validity of this test is 0.86

Statistical Analysis

For the interpretation or the analysis of data collected in the research, statistical methods were used. With the help of statistical methods perfect and scientific result can be obtained. To check difference and relation between mean score, use of statistical techniques of't' method was used.

Procedure

The study was conducted on a sample of 240 people with an HIV positive diagnosis from Ahmedabad & Bhavnagar region. The purpose of the present study was to understand the level of family and social adjustment in these individuals and to know the level of their depression. Tools used were administered on the sample.

After the collection of data 't' test was applied in order to conclude the results and interpretation of data.

RESULTS AND DISCUSSION:

The main objective of present study was to know the level of Family adjustment, Social adjustment and Depression in HIV Positive people before and after counselling. For this, statistical 't' method was used.

Results and discussion of present study are as under:

Ho_1: There will be no significant difference in Family adjustment level of HIV positive people in relation to before and after Counseling.

Table-1: Showing t-value and mean differences between before and after counselling family adjustments of HIV Positive people

Group	Family adjustment			't'
	N	M	SD	
Before Counselling	240	35.95	5.94	16.01**
After Counselling	240	46.30	8.06	

Significant level   *P < 0.05   ** P < 0.01

Table no.1 indicates that 't' test has been applied to find out whether there is any significant difference in the Family adjustment level of HIV patients before and after counselling . The calculated 't' value is found to be 16.01 which is greater than the table value and is significant at 0.01 level. Hence the null hypothesis "There will be no significant difference in Family adjustment level of HIV positive people in relation to before and after Counselling." is rejected. Therefore it is concluded that there is a significant difference between before and after counselling of HIV patients in relation to their Family adjustment. This result indicates that the mean scores for the variable of Family adjustment of before Counselling of HIV Positive were 35.95 and after Counselling were 46.30 respectively. The mean value indicates that after counselling HIV positive people have more Family Adjustment then before counselling. It means that the after Counselling HIV positive people have better family adjustment level then before counselling.

Ho_2: There will be no significant difference in Social adjustment level of HIV positive people in relation to before and after Counseling.

Table-2.: Showing t-value and mean differences between before and after counselling social adjustments of HIV Positive people

Group	Social adjustment			't'
	N	M	SD	
Before Counselling	240	36.83	6.81	11.20**
After Counselling	240	44.11	7.46	

Significant level   *P < 0.05   ** P < 0.01

Table no.2 indicates that 't' test has been applied to find out whether there is any significant difference in the social adjustment level of HIV patients before and after counselling . The calculated 't' value is found to be 16.01 which is greater than the table value and significant at 0.01 level. Hence the null hypothesis "There will be no significant difference in Social adjustment level of HIV positive people in relation to before and after Counselling." is rejected. Therefore it is concluded that there is a significant difference between before and after counselling of HIV patients in relation to their Social adjustment. This result indicates that the mean scores for the variable of Social adjustment of before Counselling of HIV Positive were 36.83 and after Counselling were 44.11 respectively. The mean value indicates that after counselling HIV positive people have more Social Adjustment then before counselling. It means that the after Counselling HIV positive people have better Social adjustment level then before counselling.

Ho₃:
There will be no significant difference in Depression of HIV positive people in relation to before and after Counseling.

Table-3.: Showing t-value and mean differences between before and after counselling Depression of HIV Positive people

Group	Depression			't'
	N	M	SD	
Before Counselling	240	159.81	15.66	14.66**
After Counselling	240	128.73	28.75	

Significant level   *P < 0.05   ** P < 0.01

Table no.3 indicates that 't' test has been applied to find out whether there is any significant difference in the Depression level of HIV patients before and after counselling . The calculated 't' value is found to be 16.01 which is greater than the table value and significant at 0.01 level. Hence the null hypothesis "There will be no significant difference in Depression level of HIV positive people in relation to before and after Counselling" is rejected. Therefore it is concluded that there is a significant difference between before and after counselling of HIV patients in relation to their Depression. This result indicates that the mean scores for the variable of Depression of before Counselling of HIV Positive was 159.81 and after Counselling was 128.73 respectively. The mean value indicates that after counselling HIV positive people have less Depression then before counselling. It means that the after Counselling HIV positive people reduce levels of Depression then before counselling .

CONCLUSION

1. HIV positive people have more Family Adjustment after counseling. It means that after counseling HIV positive people have better family adjustment level than before counseling.

2. The mean value indicates that after counseling HIV positive people have more Social Adjustment then before counseling. It means that after Counseling HIV positive people have better Social adjustment level than before counseling.

3. HIV positive people have less Depression than before counseling. It means that after Counseling HIV positive people have reduced levels of Depression then before counseling.

REFERENCES

Adam W. Carrico, Michael H. Antoni, (2008), 'Effects of Psychological Interventions on Neuroendocrine Hormone Regulation and Immune Status in HIV-Positive Persons: A Review of Randomized Controlled Trials', Psychosomatic Medicine 70, p 575-584.

Anthony Spirito, Lori J. Stark, Connie Cobiella and others, (1990), 'Social Adjustment of Children Successfully Treated for Cancer', Journal of pediatric Psychology, 15(3), p 359-371.

Antiretroviral Therapy Guidelines for HIV- Infected Adults and Adolescents Including Post-exposure Prophylaxis', (2008) NACO Ministry of Heath & Family Welfare, Government of India, p. 7-32, 54, 55, 56-65

Danie J.Repinski, Susan M. Shonk, (2002), 'Mothers and Fathers Behavior, Adolescents Self-Representation, and Adolescents Adjustment', The Journal of Early Adolescence, Vol.22, No.4, p 357-383.

Dougherty, Cynthia M., (July/August 1995), 'Psychological reactions and family Adjustment in shock versus no shock groups after implantation of internal cardioverter defibrillator', Heart & Lung: Journal of Acute & Critical Care. 24(4):281-291,.

Douglas K. Owens, Vandana Sundaram, Laura C. Lazzeroni, and other, Dec 2007, 'Prevalence of HIV Infection Among Inpatients and Outpatients in Department of Veterans Affairs Health Care Systems: Implications for Screening Programs for HIV', American journal of public health, Vol 97, No 12, p. 2173-2178.

Elizabeth A. Robinson and Linda L. Anderson. (Jun 1983), 'Family adjustment, Parental attitudes and social desirability', Journal of Abnormal Child Psychology, Vol.11, No.2, p 247-256.

Eugene W. Farber, Hamid Mirsalimi, Karen A. Williams and J. Stephen McDaniel, Dec (2003), 'Meaning of illness and Psychological Adjustment to HIV/AIDS', Psychosomatics 44, p 485-491.

Gail Ironson and H'Sien Hayward,(2008) 'Do positive Psychosocial Factors Predict Disease Progression in HIV-1? A Review of the Evidence', Psychosomatic Medicine 70, p 546-554.

Grassi, L. Pavanati, M. Cardelli R. Ferri, S. Peron, L. Jan 1999, 'HIV-risk behavior and knowledge about HIV/AIDS among patients with schizophrenia', Psychological Medicine : Volume 29(1), p 171-179.

Guidelines for Prevention and Management of Common Opportunistic Infections/ Malignancies among HIV-Infected Adult and Adolescent' p. 5-76.

HIV Counseling training modules for VCT, PPTCT and ART counselors' National Aids Control Organization, p 1-108, 151-349.

Ickovics, Jeannette R, Milan, Stephanie, Boland, and others, (Sep 2006), 'Psychological resources protect health: 5-year survival and immune function among HIV-infected women from four US cities', AIDS: Volume 20(14)11, p 1851-1860.

Ignace P. R. Vermaes, Jan R. M. Gerris and Jan M. Janssens, (2007), Parents' Social Adjustment in Families of Children with Spina Bifida: A Theory-driven Review, Journal of Pediatric Psychology, 32(10), p. 1214-1226.

Janice D. Bordeaux, Katherine A. Loveland, and others, (2003), 'Hemophilia Growth and Development Study: Caregiver Report of Youth and Family Adjustment to HIV Disease and Immunologic Compromise',Journal of pediatric psychology, Vol.28, No3, p 175-183.

Kasandariya H.V., 'A Psychological Study of Adolescent's Academic Stress and Adjustment', Ph.d. Thesis, 2008.

Kristen E. Robinson, Cynthia A. Gerhardt, Kathryn Vannatta and Robert B. Noll,'Parent and Family Factors Associated with Child Adjustment to Pediatric Cancer', Journal of Pediatric Psychology, Vol.32, No.4, p.400-410.

Lamia P. Barakat, Jennifer D. Hetzke, Bernadette Foley, and others, (2003), 'Evaluation of a Social-Skills Training Group Intervention With Children Treated for Brain Tumors: A Pilot Study', Journal of pediatric Psychology Vol, No.5, p 299-307.

Manual for Management of HIV/AIDS in children' (2004-05), NACO, IAP, UNICEF, WHO, p. 1-46, 97-125.

Michael H. A ., Kathry, E. Weaver, Suzanne C. Lechner, Neil Schneider man, 2005, 'Cognitive behavioral stress management with HIV positive homosexual men: mechanisms of sustained reductions in depressive symptoms', Chronic illness Vol 1, No.3, p 207-215.

Oyefeso A.O., Adegoke A.R., (1992), 'Psychological adjustment of Yoruba Adolescents as Influenced by family type: a research note', JOURNAL OF CHILD PSYCHOLOGY AND PSYCHIATRY AND ALLIED DISCIPLINES, May, 33(4):785-8.

Peter A. Vanable, Michal P. Carey, Donald C. Blair and Rae A. Littlewood, (Sep 2006), 'Impact of HIV-Related Stigma on Health

Behaviors and Psychological Adjustment among HIV-Positive Men and Women', AIDS and Behavior Vol 10, No.5, p 473-482.

Peter A. Wyman, J Moynihan, Shirley Eberly and others, (2007), 'Association of Family Stress with Natural Killer Cell Activity and the Frequency of illnesses in Chidern', Arch Pediatr Adolesc Med., 161(3), p 228-234.

Rachel Levy-Shiff, (2001), 'Psychological adjustment of adoptees in adulthood: Family environment and adoption-related correlates', International Journal of Behavioral Development, Vol. 25, No. 2, p 97-104 .

Rajamanickam M. (2006), 'PSYCHOLOGYCAL PERSPECTIVE OF HIV/AIDS', Concept Publishing Company, New Delhi, p 1-105.

Rise B. Goldstein, Mllory O. Johnson, and others, (2005), 'Psychological Distress, Substance Use, and Adjustment among Parents living with HIV', Chronic illness Vol 1, No.3, p 207-215.

Robin J. Jacobs, Barbara Thomlison, (2008), 'Self-Silencing and Age as Risk Factors for Sexually Acquired HIV in Midlife and Older Women', Journal of Aging and Health, Vol 1, p 120-128.

Shah. N.K., 'an Analytical Study of Marital Adjustment, Emotional Adjustment & Depression Among Working & Non Working Women', Ph.D. Thesis, 2009.

Stephen P. and Gladeana M. 'Handbook of Counseling' –Second edition, p 75-91, 421- 433.

Thakur D. (2000), 'Research Methodology in Social Sciences', Deep & Deep Publication PVT. LTD. New Delhi, p. 3-36, 101-111.

Thanulingom N. (2000-01), 'Research Methodology', Himalaya Publishing House, P 91-94, 98-102, 103-114, 142-154.

Vaghela S. , 'Study of Anxiety & Adjustment Among Executive and Non Executive Working Women, Ph.D. Thesis, 2003.

VS Helgeson, S Cohen, (March 1996),'Social support and adjustment cancer: reconciling descriptive co relational, and intervention research', Health Psychology, Vol.15, No.2. p 142-148.

Socio-Economic aspects of HIV/AIDS in Kashmir Valley

Tufail Mohammad Khoja[37], Abdul Basit Naik[38]

ABSTRACT

This research uses an economic model of risky sexual behaviour to investigate the correlation between different socio-economic attributes and HIV prevalence at district-level in Kashmir. The empirical findings show that district HIV prevalence is positively correlated to expenditure, education and the proportion of female headed households and negatively correlated to the proportion of women and their fertility. This state level HIV prevention proposes attempts to change the norms, attitudes, collective self-efficacy and risk behaviour practices in populations vulnerable to AIDS are essential for various reasons. People contract HIV as a result of sexual and drug abuse activities that take place in their day-to-day lives in the state. According to the empirical literature little attention has been given to the socio-economic context in which people live when it comes to understanding the disease. This will be preceded by a discussion of the various state engagement theories and frameworks in the context of HIV and AIDS prevention, care and support, and impact mitigation. A subsequent section will focus on the socio-economic context in relation to cultural movements and gender dynamics. The research paper will conclude with a comparison of the state engagement and socio- economic attributes and their suitability to the HIV and AIDS response among the Kashmiri people.

Keywords: HIV-AIDS, Attitude, Stigma, Kashmir, Socio-Economic Factors.

---

[37] Research Scholar RDVV Jabalpur, M.P
[38] Research Scholar MANUU Hyderabad

HIV/AIDS is one of the largest obstacles to development in many countries and is destroying the lives and livelihoods of millions of people around the world. Nearly 95 percent of all infected individuals are found in developing countries and the situation is especially problematic in Asia. India has the third largest number of people living with HIV in the world — 2.1 million at the end of 2013 — and accounts for about 4 out of 10 people living with HIV in the region. HIV is a sociocultural and socioeconomic disease in India, and the paradigm of its infection and spread particularly within the states is a reflection of the sociocultural and socioeconomic profile of the people. The factors have overlapping or interconnected relationships – none excludes the other in importance or in enhancing HIV spread and progression. These factors are further explained in the preceding discusses on the sociocultural studies. The population became aware of HIV/AIDS either from the mass media (particularly radio and television) or as usual, rumours and peer group conversations.

The presence, in the communities, of known cases of those infected with HIV/AIDS was source of information with gossips aiding in the dissemination. That none of the respondents or discussants in the BSS indicated knowledge of any HIV/AIDS victim that had been cured underscored their concept of incurability of the disease. Despite the apparent incurability of the disease, for about 70% of the single women getting pregnant was still the major concern in unprotected sex rather than HIV infection. In fact, this attitude of "one must die of something someday" is reminiscent of one caught between "the devil and the blue sea", death by hunger and death by HIV/AIDS. It further shows the societal concern regarding extramarital pregnancy – the stigma of getting an illegitimate child is paramount to the concern of contracting an infectious disease.

OBJECTIVE:

The objective of this study is to assess the socio-economic consequences of HIV/AIDS within the family.

METHODOLOGY

Different studies employ different methods to work out of the trials to get the desired objectives, but when it comes the turn of some stigmatized issues like prostitution, white slavery, lesbianism or gaiety, there always arise some ubiquitous issues. The reason behind may be that the things are linked with unethical or immoral or sometimes non-religious constructs. Same is the case with HIV/AIDS, but the difference lies in the fact that after all AIDS is a disease which has to be understood, tackled and exterminated from the life of a liver. The AIDS epidemic has posed unique challenges to the medical sciences and also for the analysis of data new statistical methods have been employed to handle such problems as the tracking and prediction of number of AIDS cases and the assessments to reach out the HIV patients and the analysis and monitoring of clinical trials with censored and missing data. So, the work will mostly base on the primary data collected from the field *plus* the quantitative and empirical techniques will be used to analyze the data. Further the work shall stand on the qualitative design as well. The historical analysis is necessary at the same time to understand the differences in the magnitude of ostracism over the last three decades. Research methodology in this changing and ever more complex environment presents great methodological changes. And so is my study depending upon.

Procedure & source of data:

Most of the estimates presented in this research are made on the basis of original analysis of available survey data. I have sought datasets from nationally representative population-based surveys in Kashmir undertaken during the 21st century. Values have been aggregated at district-level from these household surveys. The dependent variable, HIV prevalence, and the independent variables fertility and major trunk roads were already aggregated values. The empirical analysis of this thesis is mainly based on data from the Living Conditions Monitoring Survey field study and census of India (2011). This survey has a nationwide coverage on a sample basis and covers both rural and urban areas. The survey was designed to provide data on the various aspects of the living conditions of households for each and every district in Kashmir. District-level HIV prevalence are estimated figures from the Epidemiological report published in 2011, which contains epidemiological projections for the period 1985 to 2010,as I could not find proxies for mobility anywhere else. Data on adjusted total fertility rates comes from the Census of Population and Housing in 2011. Unfortunately, data on fertility rates for later years did not exist at district-level. Developing countries have a hard time gathering and updating a good database because of high costs and organization problems. High quality data is therefore a luxury article in countries like India. However, good quality data can be enhanced by using well designed questionnaires and well trained interviewers – more common when dealing with large surveys such as LCMS.

RESULTS AND DISCUSSION:

Table 1, District wise Distribution of PLWHA in Kashmir Division

Name of districts	Population 2011 census	Area [km^2]	No. of HIV patients
Kupwara	875,564	2,379	17
Anantnag	1,069,749	3,984	21
Kulgam	423,181		21
Pulwama	570,060	1,398	16
Shopian	265,960		23

Budgam	755,331	1,371	11
Srinagar	1,250,173	2,228	43
Ganderbal	297,003		9
Bandipora	385,099		5
Baramulla	1,015,503	4,588	30
Total	6,907,623	15,948	196

Source: *Field Study and Census of India 2011.*

The above table shows that maximum 22 percent of HIV patients are residing in Srinagar followed by 15 percent in Baramulla. Then comes District Shopian with 12 percent followed by District Anantnag and Kulgam both with 11 percent of HIV patients. Two more Districts Pulwama and Kupwara share a common percentile of 8 each. Three more Districts Budgam, Ganderbal, and Bandipora are having 6, 5, and 2 percent of HIV patients respectively.

J&K State is a low prevalence state where the mean prevalence rate of HIV infection among high risk groups (STD) is 0.3% and among low risk groups (ANC) is 0.04 %, as per various Sentinel Surveillance rounds conducted during last eight years. There are 2102 confirmed HIV positive cases in the State. 799 full-blown AIDS cases have been registered out of which 133 AIDS deaths have taken place so far. 518 AIDS patients including 35 children are receiving free Anti-retroviral treatment (ART) in two ART centers functioning in the State.Jammu division has highest number of HIV positive with 90% of these cases, while Kashmir with only 13% of HIV positivecasesare detected so far.

CONCLUSION

The socio-economic impact of HIV/AIDS was considerably grave, and certainly more among the sicker patients with increased severity and duration of the disease. Intensive education for PLWHAs, their family members, and other stakeholders is urgently required for the reduction of AIDS-related stigma and discrimination, as also the need for care and support. More research to get a better insight into the problem of socio-economic impact at household and community levels, and for mainstreaming of PLWHAs is the need of the hour. Services to support those affected as well as a legal framework to protect their rights is also important.

REFERENCES

Elsberg, A. & Betron, M. (2010) ' Preventing Gender-Based Violence and HIV: Lessons from the Field' AIDSTAR-One: Spotlight on Gender

India Human Development Report 2011 (Towards Social Inclusion)" (PDF). IAMR, Planning Commission, Government of India. p 257. Retrieved 5 April 2014.

Jehangir, Saleem (2013). "The AIDS Epidemic and Sociological Enquiry". Jay Kay Books.

Mbonu, N.C. et al (2009) ' Stigma of People with HIV/AIDS in Sub-Saharan Africa: A Literature Review' Journal of Tropical Medicine

Overview of HIV and AIDS in India. Retrieved from http://www.avert.org/aidsindia.htm.

Showkat A. Motta,(Dec 10, 2008) OneWorld South Asia

Sternberg, Steve (23 February 2005). "HIV scars India". USA Today.

UNAIDS (2012) ' Global Report: UNAIDS Report on the Global AIDS Epidemic 2012'

UNAIDS (2012) ' Regional Fact Sheet 2012: Asia and the Pacific'

UNAIDS (2013) ' Global Report 2013'

UNAIDS (2013) ' Global Report 2013'

UNAIDS Gap Report 2014; UNAIDS Fact Sheet 2014.

HIV/AIDS in Kashmir

Ishrat Batool Naik[39], Tejaswini Padikkal[40],

Abdul Raffie Naik[41]

ABSTRACT

AIDS is a fatal disease described variously as modern plague, scourge, distressing disease, and insidious biological disaster. It has emerged as an unprecedented pandemic cutting across all boundaries - International, Socioeconomic, Sex, Age, and Race. When people are diagnosed with HIV/AIDS, they are seen in a negative light by the people they are close to and the society at large. These factors have a lasting impact on the mental health of the people. The present study looks at the reactions the people of Kashmir, when diagnosed as being HIV positive, have faced. 50 people getting treated at an ART Center SKIMS, Soura at Srinagar were interviewed. The responses showed both positive and negative responses to the questions they were asked. This shows that HIV/AIDS people, although face the discrimination, majority of the people diagnosed as positive, have the support of family and friends and are taken care of. However, the people also face mental health issues.

Keywords: *HIV-AIDS, Social Exclusion, Kashmir*

Stigmatization of the people living with HIV/AIDS (PLWHA) can pose a significant barrier to the quality of life of a person and the health of a person. Stigma is closely related to social exclusion that could be regarded as a way of describing the discriminatory responses arising out of the process of stigmatisation. One possible reason for the social exclusion of PLWHA could be the negativity associated with the disease and the lack of information associated

---

[39] M.A, Womens Education MANUU Hyderabad
[40] Research Scholar Central University of Karnataka
[41] M.Sc. Clinical and Counselling Psychology CUK

with the spread of the disease(Fabianova, 2011). Another reason for discrimination and the stigmatization could be that people view the disease as infecting those people who deviate from the normal societal norms like homosexuals, drug users or people having multiple heterosexual partners (Habib & Rahman, 2010). The process of exclusion has been regarded as a method that has brought about in excluding the stigmatized from routine social processes.

Reading HIV/AIDS and Exclusion in Kashmir

It has been more than two decades of time that Kashmir is living with HIV/AIDS. No matter that the first case was reported in 1986, the same year that India reported its first case, HIV has not been hovering over valley the way it does in the whole of India. Fortunately the number of HIV positive patients is still very less (Around 230 according to ART cell Srinagar Report till June 2014). One of the reasons for this less number could be that people do not report the disease because of the stigma and shame that is attached with the disease. The disease has not drastically engulfed the valley, as it does as per its characteristic features and transmission. At the same time the fact cannot be overruled that Kashmir is living with this virus since 1986. Valley is suffering the way others do, but may be on smaller scale. HIV/AIDS may have least extensions in terms of Kashmir as compared to other states of the country. The question is not only what are the reasons and ways HIV AIDS spread in Kashmir, but the question why HIV could not make its avenues powerful in the valley. The main question that comes up is why is there a little number of HIV patients, even when the circumstances like illiteracy, unawareness and backwardness are in favour of transmissions and spreads? The current paper, along with the focus on the above question, will also explain the magnitude of stigma and exclusion specifically in Kashmir.

The present study is based on field study and a self-constructed questionnaire formulated on the basis of the nature of the HIV/AIDS pandemic. A well-defined section of the questionnaire is specially meant to measure the social and exclusionary aspects of the disease. Different dimensions of exclusion is separately put into course and is analysed, processed and explained by different measures like tables, charts and graphs.

Reactions of people:
When people first hear about their HIV status, they may feel shock, anger and numbness and they usually deny that they are effected by the disease. Feelings of guilt and shame are also present. People with HIV are usually stigmatized and face a lot of other problems like being looked down upon, shunned by the society as well as the family and friends. They receive little psychological and social support and are usually left to face the disease by themselves. The positive diagnosis also has a negative effect on the marital relationship wherein, the spouse usually leaves the relationship. The stigma attached with HIV usually arises from fear and lack of information about how HIV spreads and whether or not it can be controlled. This stigma leads to people facing a lot of mental health problems like depression as well as self-induced isolation leading to disrupted social relationships, thus people may not engage in any activities with people from their families, friends and society. People also have lowered self-esteem and view themselves in a negative light. There may be denial and people may also further engage in disruptive behaviours like drinking and taking drugs. This effects the quality of life of the people and also the diagnosis, disease progression and also care and may not adhere to medication, thereby letting the disease progress. Physical abuse and denial for treatment at hospitals are other issues faced by the people.

In certain cases, however, the reactions of families can be different. They may stand with and provide positive support to the effected person. This may be true of the family, friends or a spouse who stay with them and take care of the effected. The present study looks at the reactions of family and friends when they hear that the people close to them are diagnosed as being HIV positive.

Reaction of respondents diagnosed as HIV positive
Figure 1. Showing the reaction of the people on hearing about their diagnosis

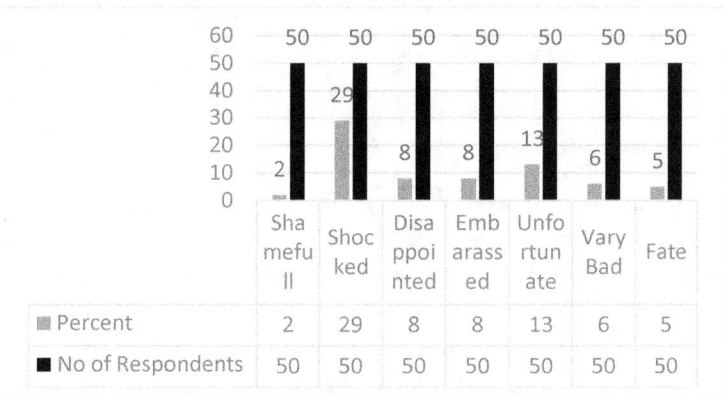

	Sha mefu ll	Shoc ked	Disa ppoi nted	Emb arass ed	Unfo rtun ate	Vary Bad	Fate
Percent	2	29	8	8	13	6	5
No of Respondents	50	50	50	50	50	50	50

Source: ART Center SKIMS Soura Srinagar.

The above graph defines the sample size of total fifty respondents. The respondents were asked about how they felt the first instance they heard about their status of being diagnosed as HIV positive. All were questioned that how they felt at the first instance when heard of their HIV positive status. 2 out of 50 respondents said they felt ashamed when came to know of their status. The maximum 58 replied that they were shocked. 16 respondents were disappointed, 26 said it was unfortunate and 16 had felt embarrassed. 12 of total said it was very bad and 6 have advocated it to fate.

Response of family members

Figure2. Showing thereaction of family members

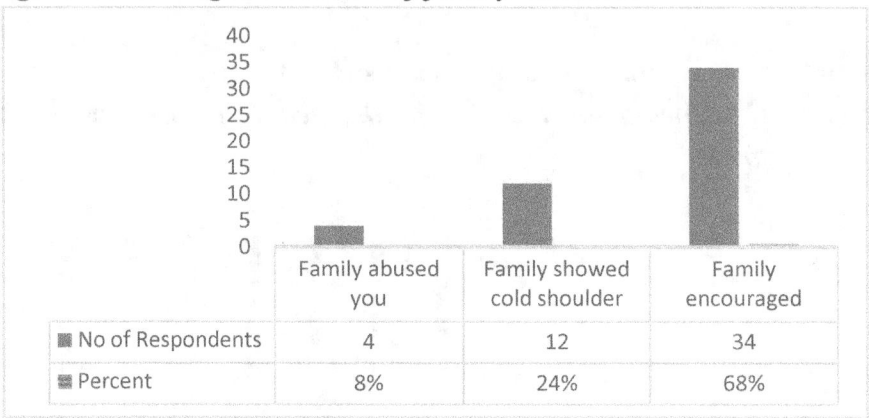

	Family abused you	Family showed cold shoulder	Family encouraged
No of Respondents	4	12	34
Percent	8%	24%	68%

Source: ART Center SKIMS Soura Srinagar.

The graph displays some interesting facts related to strength of stigma in terms of Kashmir. It shows quite well that 68 % of respondents say that they have been encouraged and taken care of since they were tested positive. 24 % said that some of the family members started to show a cold shoulder as they are afraid of what will happen if they come into contact with a person diagnosed as being HIV positive. The very least 8 % of the people replied in affirmative when asked if they were abused sometimes being HIV positive.

Effect on marital relationship
Figure3. Showing the reaction of the Spouse

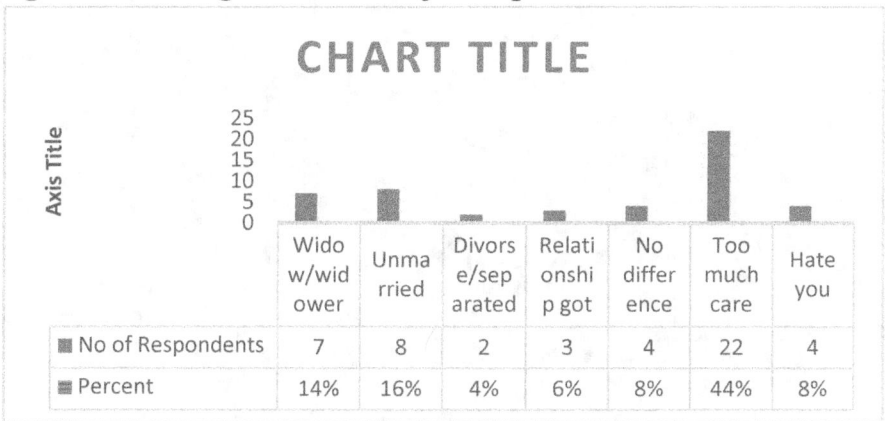

CHART TITLE	Wido w/wid ower	Unma rried	Divors e/sep arated	Relati onshi p got	No differ ence	Too much care	Hate you
No of Respondents	7	8	2	3	4	22	4
Percent	14%	16%	4%	6%	8%	44%	8%

Source: ART Center SKIMS Soura Srinagar.

The graph clearly defines the reaction of spouse when getting to know the HIV status of his/her spouse. 14% of respondents are already widow are widower and 16% of all are unmarried. The remaining 70 % have many different things to say. The majority of 44% says that their spouses started to take much care of them. Although 8% says their husband/wife started to dislike him/her and the same percentage says that there was no difference in relationship at all. Six percent says that relationship got deteriorated and four % people's marriages saw the drastic outcome in the form of divorce or separation.

Reaction of friends

Figure 4. Showing the reaction of friends

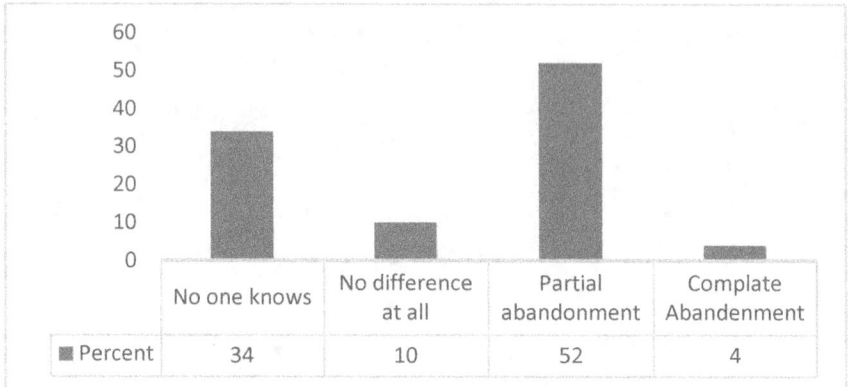

Percent	No one knows	No difference at all	Partial abandonment	Complate Abandenment
	34	10	52	4

Source: ART Center SKIMS Soura Srinagar.

The above graph shows the identification of the fact of stigma which is attached to HIV and AIDS. The close friends may get detached after their friend has been declared HIV positive. 42 % of the respondents experienced the partial abandonment from their close mates and friends. The major reason for this may be the fear of transmission of HIV. The friends will continue to love and take care of their HIV positive friends but at the same time they keep themselves at back foot when need to come closer. The ten % say that was not a prominent change in such relationships as in before and after. A very less % say that they experienced complete abandonment from their friends. There is one more important thing to identify here that thirty % of HIV positive persons are still hiding their HIV status to their close and intimate friends.

The bar charts show a much expected numbers as most of the people in Kashmir believe that people diagnosed as HIV positive are just like others who suffer other diseases like diabetes, blood pressure, cancer etc. but this can be somewhat on humanitarian grounds. Most of the people seem to have no complaints with the HIV positive persons but they surly seem to part from such people as well taking their own health statuses in to considerations. Some of the respondents say the people take this epidemic otherwise and incorrect. They seemingly put a bad tag on it and hence People living with HIV/AIDS do suffer by the same. Only a small number of people say that people, on knowing their status, make bitter faces and show resentment towards them. Here it is further to note that most of respondents have kept their health status a secret even from the close relatives. Such people mostly experience self-stigma.

Reaching health centers and difficulties thereof
Figure 5. Showing discrimination faced in Hospitals.

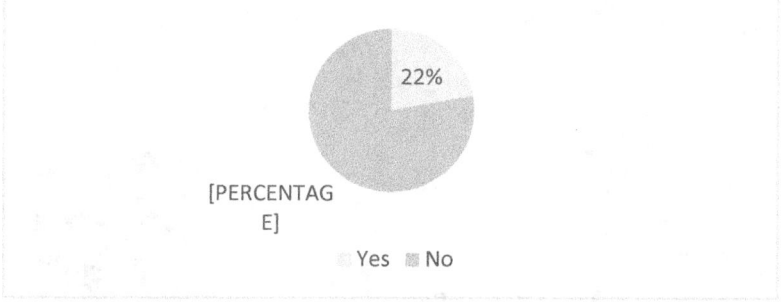

Source: ART Center SKIMS Soura Srinagar.

The pie chart shows that the intensity of care and treatment by the medical faculty. 78 % of the respondents admit that they do not face any complications from the medical faculty while availing the medical facilities. About 22 % somehow where not happy with the facilities for the reason they are supposed to visit the ART center Srinagar each month to get a month's long medication course. There are some very poor who cannot afford even the bus fare. For such reasons they seemed unhappy with the medical administration and government policies. The medical staff along with the patients feel the necessity for more ART centers in Kashmir.

Impact of disease (HIV/AIDS) on mental state

HIV seems to have an impact on human beings. The disease alters the course of life of people by creating uncertainty, disturbance, imbalance and chaos to life. During the interview, people stated that they felt broken and started crying. As most of the Kashmiris are Muslims and are believers and god-fearing, they said that they spend most of the time remembering God and in prayers repenting their ill-doings. Most of the people also stated that the disease felt like a 'death-sentence'.

Figure 6. Showing HIV/AIDS and mental condition

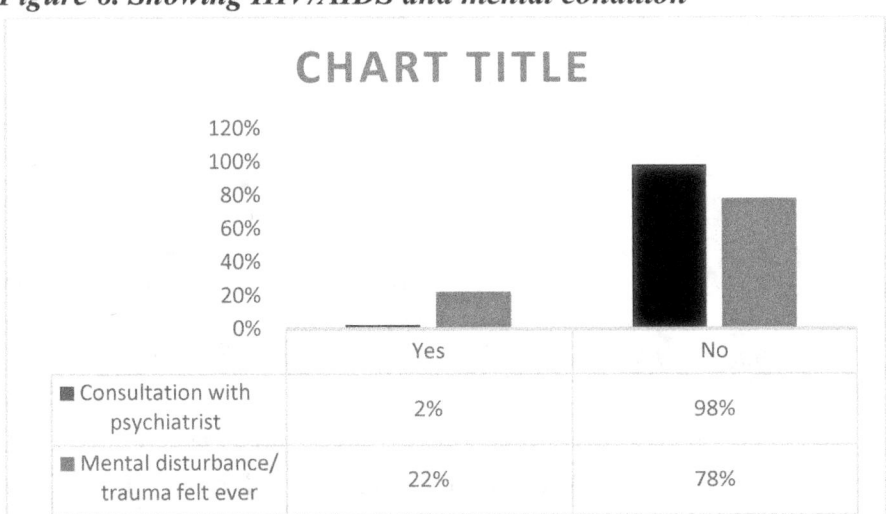

CHART TITLE

	Yes	No
■ Consultation with psychiatrist	2%	98%
■ Mental disturbance/ trauma felt ever	22%	78%

Source: ART Center SKIMS Soura Srinagar.

The respondents were asked two questions. One was if the patient felt any kind of mental disturbance or trauma of any sort. Seventy eight percent of respondents replied in thaaffirmative and twenty two percent of them replied in the negative. This shows that HIV has an impact on the mental condition of the person. The second question asked was whether they had consulted a psychiatrist ever. Only two percent of the people said yes and the rest ninety eight percent of people said no for this question. This shows that people do not feel the need to go to a psychiatrist or are unaware about the benefit of going to a psychiatrist.

CONCLUSION

Kashmir sees the inflow of thousands of armed forces and labourers coming from different regions and diverse backgrounds as well as there is an increasing movement of Kashmiris to other areas of India where they might indulge in high risk behaviour (Mir, Sofi, Ahmad, Dar, Ahmad & Siddeque, 2010). During late eighties the HIV/AIDS pandemic saw its way in to Kashmir. There are still many ways through which the disease spreads. For example intravenous Drug Users (IDU), and Unprotected Sex (US) have been the major factors for the transmission of HIV in the valley. Further the majority of the people views the epidemic as a disease of people who do not follow the norms of the society. Many people refuse to get treated as the diagnosis is associated with shame and disgust and the people are unaware about the spread of the disease.

HIV/AIDS is a one name to sufferings, stigma, hatred, ostracism, discrimination, exclusion and more. It has become a universal phenomenon and results in an enormous human suffering and deaths. It is no more an exaggeration that people fear of HIV/AIDS death less than its social implications. Its reach and effect cuts across all dimensions of society causing instability to human security.

REFERENCES

Jehangir, S. (2013). *The AIDS epidemic and sociological enquiry*. Srinagar, Jay Kay books.

Fabianova, L. (2011). Psychosoical aspects of people living with HIV/AIDS. In G. Letamo (Ed.), *Social and Psychological Aspects of HIV/AIDS and their Ramifications*. InTech. Retrieved from http://www.intechopen.com/books/social-and-psychological-aspects-of-hiv-aids-and-their-ramifications/psychosocial-aspects-of-people-living-with-hiv-aids

Habib, T. Z., & Rahman, M. S. (2010). Psycho-Social Aspects of AIDS as a Chronic Illness: Social Worker Role Perspective. *Antrocom: Online Journal of Anthropology, 6*(1), 79–89.

Mir, M.A., Sofi, F.A., Ahmad, S.N., Dar, M.R., Ahmad, P.M., Siddeque, M,A. (2010). Clinical and demographic profile of HIV/AIDS patients diagnosed at a tertiary care centre in Kashmir. *Journal of Pakistan medical association.*101-109.

Iqbal, M. (2015). HIV/AIDS and Social Exclusion in Kashmir. hyderabad, Telangana, india.IIPS/ORC Marco: National Family Health Survey of India 1998-99(2002). NFHS-2; J& K, October, p. 149-55

Acknowledgment

Official Partners

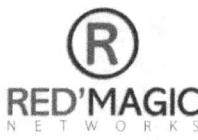 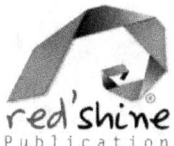 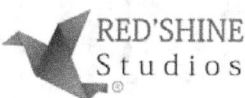 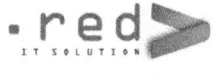

Family Partners

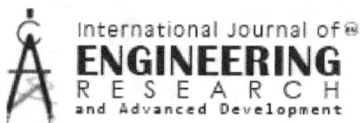 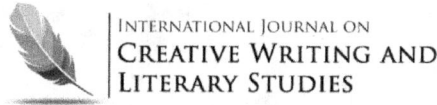

Library Partners

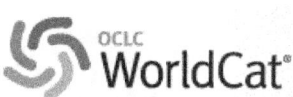

WZB

TIB | GERMAN NATIONAL LIBRARY OF SCIENCE AND TECHNOLOGY

APAIS Thesaurus
National Library of Australia

Publisher Partners

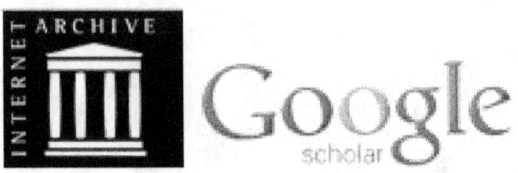

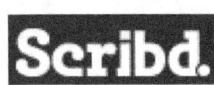
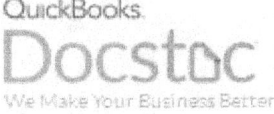
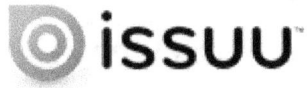

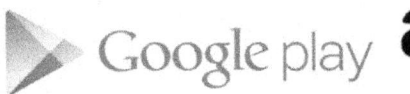

Special Issue Publishing Partners